Brace for Impact

Coping with Post Traumatic Stress Disorder

Joseph E. Panko, Jr.
with Trish Stukbauer

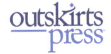

Brace for Impact
Coping with Post Traumatic Stress Disorder
All Rights Reserved.
Copyright © 2024 Joseph E. Panko, Jr.
v3.0 r1.0

The opinions expressed in this manuscript are solely the opinions of the author and do not represent the opinions or thoughts of the publisher. The author has represented and warranted full ownership and/or legal right to publish all the materials in this book.

This book may not be reproduced, transmitted, or stored in whole or in part by any means, including graphic, electronic, or mechanical without the express written consent of the publisher except in the case of brief quotations embodied in critical articles and reviews.

Outskirts Press, Inc.
http://www.outskirtspress.com

Paperback ISBN: 978-1-9772-6286-8
Hardback ISBN: 978-1-9772-7215-7

Cover & Interior Images © 2024 Joseph Panko. All rights reserved - used with permission.

Outskirts Press and the "OP" logo are trademarks belonging to Outskirts Press, Inc.

PRINTED IN THE UNITED STATES OF AMERICA

Dedication

To my wonderful wife Susan

and our parents

Bob and Cathy Adams,

and Joe and Olga Panko

---◆---

Special Thanks to

Joseph Bertolami

Dr. Edward Craighead

Delcy Ziac Fox

Edward J. Hatch, Jr.

Dr. Ranga Krishnan

Jim Nantz, CBS Sports

Jason Orello

Charlie Williams

Table of Contents

About the Author	i
What Readers are Saying	iii
Foreword	v
Introduction – Meet Mary	vii
Chapter 1 – What is Post Traumatic Stress Disorder?	1
Chapter 2 – The Plane Crash	4
Chapter 3 – Birth of a Salesman and Childhood Traumas	20
Chapter 4 – The Believers Club	36
Chapter 5 – Lasting Friendships	77
Chapter 6 – Family and Friends	92
Chapter 7 – Techniques for Coping – The Puzzle Principle	96
Chapter 8 – Faith Can Move Mountains	108
Chapter 9 – Positive Perseverance	111
Appendix – PTSD Resources	114

About the Author

I am grateful for the many experiences and educational opportunities provided by my mother and father. I've had the chance to be somewhat successful in professional bowling and also had the good fortune to be a third-generation IBM employee. I had many experiences that were successful in achieving the goals laid out by my executive management at IBM. Being married 50 years to my wonderful wife Susan has given me an opportunity to learn patience and to be a team player working toward a great life with my best friend.

What Readers are Saying

Brace for Impact is a gripping account of Joe Panko's experience as a survivor of USAir Flight emergency landing in the East River in New York City. Despite surviving the crash, Panko found himself struggling with post-traumatic stress disorder (PTSD) in the aftermath. In this book, Panko courageously shares his journey of healing and finding hope after such a traumatic event. By sharing his story, Panko offers a message of inspiration and a roadmap for others who may be battling PTSD. With raw honesty and vulnerability, **Brace for Impact** is a story of courage, resilience, and the power of the human spirit to overcome adversity.

- K. Ranga Rama Krishnan, MD

Joe Panko is a kind-hearted friend who lives to help others. **Brace for Impact** will help countless people navigate life's ups and downs.

Bravo my friend!

P.S. So much of it I never knew.

- Jim Nantz, CBS Sports

Within the context of an unexpected and life-changing event, Joe Panko details a compelling and engaging account of his coping with the associated trauma. Panko was going about his business, having been a successful professional bowler and now a third-generation IBM employee. This all changed in a few seconds as the plane on which he was a passenger failed to take off but rather broke into pieces as it slid into the East River beside LaGuardia Airport. Coping with the impact of pain and trauma from witnessing death and despair that night required that he grow from within and find ways to enhance meaning in his life. As you read this stimulating book, you will discover a genuinely kind, uniquely generous, and extremely funny and humorous person, who describes relationships and their impact on his and other's lives so accurately, you will become a member of his "believers club." In coping with trauma, Panko has found a way to draw upon his seemingly unending friendships to bring good to others, allowing both his friends and himself to bring hope and joy to thousands of unsuspecting children. Far removed from his entertaining entrepreneurship of elementary school and now in the Fall of his life, he shares in powerful and emotional stories, his coping experiences with others who might have suffered trauma, so they, like he, might find success in living life in fuller and more meaningful ways.

- W. Edward Craighead, Ph.D., ABPP Professor, Emory University

There are different forms of PTSD, whether it's as a civilian or military. Joe has figured out what works for him. It could work for you.

- Jason Morello, Staff Sergeant First Class, US Army Special Forces

You will cry! You will laugh! More importantly, you will realize that you can do something to make someone's life better.

- Charlie Williams, Colonel, U.S. Army, West Point Graduate

Foreword

Brace for Impact has given me an opportunity to share my challenges and successes in combating Post Traumatic Stress Disorder (PTSD). Many of us have achieved multiple successes, but also have faced many challenges due to losses we have experienced in our lives. This book gives readers an opportunity to look at various ideas that might help them face and overcome those challenges.

In the pages of this book, I have the chance to share many of my experiences with professional athletes, actors, actresses, and medical folks who have given me the opportunity to share their talents and, in doing so, to raise money for charities across the country. Giving gifts and inspirational items to those in need has been an essential part of my PTSD recovery. The look of joy and the friendship I have received from so many over the years has been most helpful, not only for my own recovery, but for others as well.

It is my hope that the structure of this book gives the reader an opportunity to reflect on personal successes and offers tangible solutions for processing tragedies.

Introduction – Meet Mary

Trauma takes many forms. Sometimes, it hits you with the blunt force of a plane crash. Other times, it's the subtle silence of a small child who has seen and felt far too much for her years. That was the case with Mary.

As I was making my rounds through a Charlotte hospital some years ago and dropping off toys for abused and very ill children, I stopped by the nurse's station. On my mind and in my hands was a special doll, and I needed the right little girl to give it to. Now this doll was far from ordinary; first of all, she was huge, plus, she did just about everything except wash your dishes for you. The nurse immediately said, "Mary. She's been here for about a week and a half now, and she hasn't said a word. We can't get her to talk, and she hardly eats anything."

As with all the children in that ward and in the hospital, I wasn't privy to the details of her situation for privacy reasons. The staff couldn't tell me what had happened to her, all I could see were the results. And in this case, her situation had robbed her of her will to connect with others.

I walked into Mary's room with the nurse, saw a young girl of about eight years old and introduced myself. "Hi, I'm Joe. I'm here to see how you are doing, and I got you this present." When she saw the doll, her eyes opened wide, but she didn't say a word.

Lunch arrived and as they set it down in front of her, I asked, "Are you ready to eat something?" She just looked at me blankly, didn't say anything, and didn't make a move toward her plate. I walked toward her plate and said, "This looks like you've got a great lunch here. You've got chicken. You've got peas, and you've got mashed potatoes. Do you like your chicken, peas and mashed potatoes?" She looks up at me and shakes her head a very slow, no. I saw my opening. "I see exactly why. You've got to mix the peas with the mashed potatoes. If you put the peas by themselves – yuck," I said as I made my best disgusted face. "They are terrible on their own. You've got to mix them." So, I mixed them and grabbed the spoon, tasted it, and said, "So much better. Now you taste it." She actually took her fork and tried some, so I asked, "How is it?" She shakes her head no again. So, I said, "Well try it again, maybe you got too many peas and not enough potatoes on that spoon." She tries it again and ends up eating another mouthful.

After she gets those few bites in her and loses interest in her food again, I tell her: "I brought this dolly, because I know you're going to get better. When you go home, you get to take the dolly home with you." There was no reaction from Mary, so I kept talking, "It's for you to keep." I explained that she could change her clothes, comb her hair that looked just like her own pretty hair, and I went on and on about all the things this dolly could do. She still didn't react, so I put the dolly in her arms, and as I turned to walk away, she said, "Thank you mister."

Well, you would have thought a bomb went off in that room. The nurse who was watching the whole thing was in shock. She yelled for the doctors, two of whom came running in. I replied, "You are welcome, Mary. That dolly is for you. Do you have other dollies?" Then she actually answered, "Yes, but not as nice as this one." From there, she started talking to me about her other dolls, and I after a while, I asked if she was going to finish her lunch. She replied, "Yeah, I'm pretty hungry." I said, "Well, don't forget to mix your peas with your mashed potatoes," So she mixes up more, and starts taking a few bites, so I urge, "Don't forget that chicken." And she started working on her chicken. By this point, I was really starting to lose it as I watched this little girl who had been so withdrawn from life that she did not want to speak or eat begin the road back to recovery – all because of a random gift from a stranger.

Helping Mary and countless other children and adults like her through the years is why I give back after my own traumatic injuries sustained during a highly publicized plane crash and through many all-too-common episodes in my own life. The seemingly simple act of giving back not only gave me the will to go on, but the act itself gives so many others the will to overcome as well.

What follows is my journey. My hope is that it provides steps for others to follow or leads you to blaze your own path.

After surviving the plane crash at La Guardia, Joe Panko was happy to be back in his own bed.

Then the hurricane hit.

It was a tough week for Joe Panko.

On Wednesday, September 20, the jet in which he was a passenger skidded off a runway at La Guardia and into the East River.

Fortunately, Joe escaped with only minor injuries and was able to fly home to Concord the next day.

Joe reached his home later that evening and tucked himself into bed. Then, at about 4 a.m. on Friday, Hurricane Hugo rolled through town, damaging Joe's house and property.

Through all this, Joe considers himself a lucky man.

This is Joe. At his insurance agent's.

"As I woke up on Thursday, I had survived a plane crash. As I woke up on Friday, I had survived a hurricane. However, there was a lot of damage to my property."

We started processing Joe's claim the following day at our Emergency Claims Center, and by Monday, SAFECO Claims Specialist Larry Ellis was inspecting the damage to Joe's property.

"The way the process was set up, it was obvious that SAFECO wanted to see that claims got the attention they needed and people did not have to wait," says Joe.

Within days, Joe received a check from SAFECO covering the damage left by Hugo.

True, Joe's story is a bit unusual. But in hundreds of other claims left in the wake of Hurricane Hugo, the conclusion is the same: fast, efficient service by concerned SAFECO agents and claims adjusters.

If this is the kind of service you expect from your insurance company, we suggest you call one of the independent SAFECO agents listed below.

You might even sleep a little better at night. We know Joe is.

SAFECO

CHAPTER 1

What is Post Traumatic Stress Disorder?

You have PTSD. That phrase has become almost too common in our world today. Initially used almost exclusively when talking about the military, Post-Traumatic Stress Disorder has been tossed around in pop culture to encompass a wide range of conditions and myriad issues.

By the book, PTSD is defined as a mental health problem that some people experience after a life-threatening event. Those events can range from surviving military combat to living through a natural disaster, a horrific car accident, or a physical or sexual assault. Sometimes, you don't have to live through the event yourself – seeing it at close range can be enough to trigger PTSD. Just think of the impact that the death of a loved one or the suicide of a friend or family member can have, or the trauma experienced by a child who witnesses a sibling being abused.

In my case, it was a 1989 plane crash into New York's East River that triggered PTSD.

After any of these events, experts say that it is normal to feel on edge, to have upsetting memories, or to have difficulty sleeping. People impacted by PTSD may have difficulty resuming normal routines, coping with work or school, or even enjoying the activities they used to love.

In people who don't develop PTSD, these symptoms gradually decrease over time. Sometimes, they don't show up immediately but manifest months or even years after the initial experience, but they do fade over time.

For someone who has PTSD, that's not necessarily the case. They can have flashbacks that make them feel as if they are reliving the event, terrifying nightmares, severe anxiety, and uncontrollable thoughts about the event. They can experience dramatic negative mood swings, and physical and emotional reactions to any reminders of the trauma. These symptoms go far beyond "normal" coping mechanisms and interfere with daily living – and they last for a minimum of 6 months up to years after the event.

Anyone can be impacted by PTSD; it's not something that you choose or a sign of mental, physical, or emotional weakness. There are, however, some factors that make it more likely that an individual will experience PTSD.

Of course, there's the trauma that starts it, which is unfortunately all too common. By some estimates, about 50% of women in the United States and 60% of men will experience the level of trauma necessary to trigger PTSD at some point in their lifetimes. According to the U.S. Department of Veteran's Affairs, which understandably has an exceptional grasp of the subject, approximately 7 or 8 out of every 100 people who experience this type of trauma will develop PTSD, and about 8 million adults have PTSD during any given year.

So, what it is that pushes that 7% over the proverbial edge?

There are lots of numbers and statistics that medical experts can point to. Women are more than twice as likely to be impacted as men. Adults aged

18-24 seem more vulnerable than those who are older. The National Institute of Mental Health mentions some risk factors that begin to dig a little deeper into the heart of the issue. Contributing factors include the person getting physically hurt in the event, seeing another person get hurt or seeing a dead body, having experienced childhood trauma, feeling helpless or fearful during the event, and dealing with stress afterward.

In my own case, it was all those factors.

Other factors that I didn't experience but which also can contribute are having a lack of social and family support after the trauma or having a history of mental illness or substance abuse.

If left untreated, PTSD can lead to suicidal thoughts, and ultimately action. That's why it is so vital that anyone who is experiencing these symptoms seek professional help to get them through it and develop a positive coping strategy to carry them through what may be rough days ahead.

In my own case, I was fortunate enough to have both some of the best professional help you can get and a passion for making children smile that led me to what I feel in many ways is my life's work. My journey from my first incident of childhood trauma to brushes with fame, material success in sports and business, the plane crash that triggered my PTSD, and eventually finding my calling as a way to cope with it all was long and winding.

It is my hope that sharing my story may help others recognize the signs of PTSD in themselves or someone they love and shorten their path toward recovery.

Need help right now?
The National Suicide Prevention Hotline is available 24/7 at no charge and offers live assistance in English, Spanish and for the deaf or hard of hearing.
You can reach them at 988.

CHAPTER 2

The Plane Crash

In 1989 I had a wonderful job at IBM as a Manager of Worldwide Financial Planning for the banking business, the insurance business, and part of the corporation's software business, not only domestically, but around the world. The banking products were made in Charlotte and Raleigh, North Carolina. In the late 1980s, the doctors in our Raleigh laboratory came up with the SKU that we use for products now. We thought that every product would one day have a SKU number, and today it certainly does. But my job at the time was financial planning and reporting regarding these particular products.

As we sometimes did, we were flying from Charlotte to New York for a meeting on Monday of that fateful week. We'd been working for quite a number of months on a particular product that we were selling to another large domestic company. It was a particular part of the banking business that we were going to sell to that organization. There was a lot of information that was needed about the past progress of this particular product, the current progress this product was making in the laboratory, and how the product was progressing to be used in the marketplace.

We were working that Monday, Tuesday, and some of Wednesday, and finally, our analysis and our presentation was ready to give to the Chairman of IBM, who was John Akers at the time. Our division president, Bill Bowles, was an early bird. I'm not sure he slept for a total of three hours a day. Bill was a very outgoing executive for IBM and a very personable gentlemen, but he always wanted to have early meetings. As we concluded Tuesday's meeting, he said, "See you tomorrow morning at 6:30." That meant I'd have to get up at 5:00 a.m. to grab a little something for breakfast, shower and the like, and be ready for the meeting. This particular day was going to be a long one, because we were to meet the chairman in the afternoon. We met Bill at 6:30, which meant promptly at 6:30 a.m. and you had better not be late, and we weren't. We laid out our plan with our presentation, charts, and other items that we had ready for the chairman. As was typical, we had numerous views of the plan that day before we got to the chairman.

The stressful part of this assignment had to do with the levels in the corporation whom we were seeing that day. Seeing the chairman always came with some anticipation and stress. There was always some normal anxiety about how the chairman was going to react to a particular plan. It was important to have all our ducks in a row. What's interesting is that I had a team of financial analysts who worked with me that day. They had never met the chairman. When I told them that they were going to meet him, they responded that I would, but they wouldn't, because they were at a lower level. I had them in a waiting room, and I went to the chairman personally, and said, "I'd really like to introduce you to the team that put this information together." He said he would be glad to do so. He came by and I had the opportunity to introduce them all. They were amazed that I got that accomplished, because when you say you're going to meet somebody of that particular level in any corporation, there's always some excitement in that.

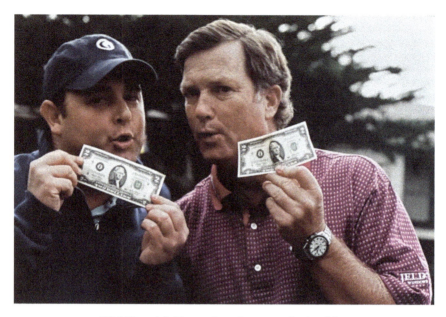

$2 bills with Peter Jacobson and a buddy.

With that, we went through the big meeting, which was very successful, and then headed home. Because of my level in the company, I typically wouldn't get to ride in a corporate limousine, but we had a limousine that night to take us to LaGuardia International, where we were catching a flight home to Charlotte. It was raining that evening, and we weren't necessarily late, but we also couldn't dawdle if we wanted to get to the airport on time. We got to the airport, and I had a gentleman help me with my bag. I gave him my last $2 bill. I'd been carrying $2 bills since I was 14 years old. I really didn't think about that fact that I gave him my last $2 bill until afterward. In any case, he helped me with my bag. We got checked in at the airport and got to the gate only to find out that our flight was delayed.

We progressed to the USAir Club, where we could sit and talk about the successes of the day. I was with Jerry Holmes, the controller of our banking division, and he and I were flying back to Charlotte together. There were other IBM employees with us on the plane, but they were in New York for different marketing business versus what we were doing. As we kept an eye on the flight schedule, our 8:00 p.m. flight was delayed until 8:30 p.m. We decided to stay in the USAir Club and go down when the 8:30 flight started to board. The flight was delayed until 9:00 p.m., and then delayed again until 9:30, and then delayed again until 10:00. At 10:00 p.m., they canceled the flight.

As we searched for options, we discovered a flight at the gate across the aisle that was heading to Greensboro, North Carolina. We were able to get on the flight to Greensboro, only to discover that our flight to Charlotte was reopened again. There were evidently two flights that were scheduled to go to Norfolk, Virginia, that evening. Someone realized that didn't make any sense and decided that they'd take flight A and reroute it to Charlotte, while flight B would go to Norfolk. We played a bit of gate roulette, asking the gate attendants to be certain that we were booked on the new flight to Charlotte before they canceled our seats on the flight to Greensboro.

In the end, we got on the flight to Charlotte, which changed my life. The flight had been renamed Flight 5050, leading to a joke that I would make for years about having a 50/50 shot of survival on that trip. What happens as I understand it is that when a flight gets canceled, it gets reassigned a new number from a list. Flight 49 was used, so we became flight 50.

When Jerry and I boarded the plane on that rainy night, we both got aisle seats in Row 18. Jerry was in 18C, and I was an 18D. Fortunately, since it was a made-up flight, we had more room to spread out. I was exhausted. It was now about 10:30 p.m., and I was really looking forward to getting home. I buckled up and took my shoes off. I had a new pair of shoes at the time, because of course, when you're seeing the chairman, you've got to get new shoes, new socks, new underwear, the whole thing. My glasses were bothering me, so I took them off and put them in my shoes so I wouldn't lose them.

I was starting to drift to sleep when we finally got the clearance to get ready to fly. We were backed up maybe 15 airplanes, so we were waiting on the tarmac for 10 or 15 minutes, and I started dozing off pretty badly.

It was now after 11:20 p.m., and the plane was cleared for takeoff. When we started to take off at 11:29 p.m., I was leaning back in my seat, almost reclined. The Boeing 737 started to take off, and it seemed as if it was taking off and taking off and taking off without getting up in the air. I thought for just a fraction of a second, "We should be up by now." As soon as I had that thought, the pilot reversed the engines and seemingly slammed on the brakes. I sat up straight and yelled to Jerry, "Put your head down!" I remember putting my head down. The plane carrying 61 passengers flew off the wet runway and crashed into the East River, where it broke apart. When the plane hit the water, my seat broke. I was thrown into the seat in front of me, and I was knocked out.

I don't recall what happened after the impact, but I was unconscious for what I later estimated to be 30 to 45 minutes. When I came to, water was up to my chest. That was probably what woke me up. It was September 20, so the water wasn't really cold, but it certainly wasn't warm either. With the water level all the way up to my chest, I think it revived me.

I looked up and down the aisles of the plane and there was nobody there. Because I was hungry, it had been a long day, I was in shock, and I have a crazy sense of humor, I yelled out, "What? I missed dinner?" That initial reaction was to become a point of interest for my psychiatric team in the future.

Since there was no one there to help, I unbuckled and tried to stand up. Before I did that, I frantically looked for my shoes, putting my hands down in the dark water. I couldn't find my shoes or my glasses;

both had floated away. If you listen to the safety speech at the beginning of every flight, they always talk about the emergency lights in the floor and how they are supposed to light up, but there was no light at all on this night. The only light I could see was at the door, and I saw a figure standing there. I wasn't sure whether it was Jerry or whether it was an angel saying to me, "Joe! Joe! Come out this way." There was the glow of a light on the other side of that door. I don't know whether that light was from the runway or the rescue efforts, but that was the only light I could see.

I stood up, unsure what had happened other than the fact that I was in the plane in the water. There was one of the emergency windows that pushed out on my left-hand side several aisles away. Barefoot, I walked toward it, holding onto the seats to the left and right of me as I walked. I stepped outside to find about 8 or 10 people on the wing holding a rope. Evidently there's a rope that progresses from the door for the length of the wing to help hold you up if you find yourself in the water. It is worth noting that none of the oxygen masks came down. People didn't seem to have their seat cushions with them for flotation purposes. But neither did I. I was first of all in shock, but primarily just interested in getting out of the plane as quickly as possible.

As I stepped up from the floor of the plane onto the wing, I found a lady holding a baby, some other people, and Jerry at the other end of the wing holding on to the rope. As I stood up on the wing and I got my bearings, I saw that there was fuel spilled from the plane everywhere on the surface of the water. There were people on the runway looking down at us, and I started yelling to them in my shock and panic. I yelled, "I'm going to swim. It's going to blow up!" They said, "No, it's not going to blow up. You'll be safe." I kept yelling, "I know it's gonna blow up. It's gonna blow up. Get us out of here." They kept trying to reassure me and when I finally calmed down a bit, I yelled, "Ok so we got 3 who say it's going to blow up and another 3 who say it's not. What do you think?" Nobody said anything, but they were probably all looking at me and thinking, "Who is this jerk?"

Pretty quickly after I concluded that I wasn't going to swim and did verify that Jerry was in fact on the wing, the lady who was holding the baby started yelling "Help!" She had lost her footing and was slipping down the wing. I grabbed onto her and started pulling her back up. Well, as I did that, I started to slip down the wing toward the water. I was able to push her toward the center of the wing and helped prevent her and her baby from going into the water. Then the team that had the rope gave me more slack to grab onto, and I was able to pull myself back up on the wing.

As I was standing on the wing waiting for help to arrive to take us to shore, Jerry said "Joe, can you get to my briefcase?" Remember, I was the closest one to the door. I said, "I think so," and I went back in the plane. I was probably somewhere around Aisle 10, which was about 15 feet or so away from where his briefcase was. I inched down a few feet and then down a few more feet but the water seemed at that point to be all the way up to the top of the aisles. So, I came back out, and said, "No, I don't think I can get to your briefcase." Jerry said, "What about my jacket? Can you get my jacket? It's got my Bible in it." So, I went back into the plane a second time, again in shock, and saw something that would haunt me for years – the bodies of two women who had been seated near the rear of the plane. At the time, I didn't think twice about going back in, again probably due to my shock. Here my boss was saying, to misquote Don Rickles. "Here's your cookie. Eat your cookie. If you get my jacket, you get two cookies."

As I walked back down the aisle, the plane shifted three feet. Water that had been up to my knees was all of sudden up to my chin. I could have sworn that somebody was at the door, saying "Sir, get back out of the plane," or maybe I just realized how much I needed to get out of that situation. In either case, I backed out carefully, got back on the wing and told Jerry I couldn't reach his jacket, but I was sure that they would be able to salvage it for him.

At that point, a rubber rescue raft floated by, and Jerry said, "Joe, come this way." The other people on the wing were just standing there, looking at the rescue folks on the runway, watching things going on around them, but not really paying attention to the fact that they were standing on a wing right by the rescue boat. Looking back on it, I realize that they also were in shock. But I knew I had to get off that wing. So, I passed by people, walking behind them as they were holding on to the rope, holding onto their shoulders, and saying "excuse me" at every turn. I went from point A to point R to get into that rubber raft with Jerry, because the folks on the wing, between me and it, weren't paying any attention. We both got into the raft with some others. Unfortunately, the person driving the raft said, "I'm going to take you over to the rescue boat." The boat was on the right side of the airplane and the raft was on the left side. Once we got to the proper place, we realized that the raft was about 12' below the boat, and no one had any idea how to move us from one to the other. Meanwhile, our raft navigator went to another area to try to pick a couple other people out of the water. However, the process of pulling them aboard was making the rubber raft unsteady. I said to him, "Why don't you just take us to shore and come back and get these people?" He goes, "Ahh, good idea." Some other guy in the rubber raft responds, "No shit!" We were all in shock. We had just survived a plane crash and this navigator is blundering around like he's got nothing better to do on a Wednesday night.

With that decision, we progressed toward the shore where the Port Authority building was, and we reached a boat launch area where there was a ramp. The driver pulled the raft in as closely as he could, but we had to get out of the raft and into the water again to make it to shore. So, after drying out for some period of time, I was back in water up to my chest again. Fortunately, I was able to walk from the ramp into the Port Authority building where there were medical people attending to us.

When you have an accident of any kind, you want to call your loved ones. I saw a payphone on the wall, and because I had an IBM phone card – remember, this was before cell phones, I was able to quickly use it to call my wife Susan. It was probably about 1:00 a.m. at this point. When she answered the phone, I told her that I wasn't going to be able to get home that night. She asked if I was okay or if I had car trouble or more meetings. I said, "I'm sure the car is fine, but Suzi, I just survived a plane crash. I don't know how bad I am. I'm really not feeling too well, but I'm okay at this point. Turn on the news and you should be able to see what happened. Once I find out more, I'll call you."

Fortunately for Susan, her parents were visiting from California at the time, so she wasn't alone in the house when she heard the news. They all got up to watch CNN and saw the plane in the water and actually saw some footage of me on the wing. Elsewhere, my aunt was ironing and watching Johnny Carson. They broke into the Johnny Carson show to show the plane crash. She looked at the TV and said, "My goodness, there's Joseph on the wing!" I was able to use my phone card so that Jerry could talk to his wife, Paula, and assure her that he was also okay. She also tuned into to see him on CNN.

At that point, medical people came to me and asked me a bunch of questions. I told them that I really couldn't feel my legs very well, and that it was getting worse as I sat there. They asked if I had experienced back problems in the past, and I reassured them that while I had, they were nothing like the extensive pain I was now experiencing. They put me on a backboard, securing my neck, and they tied me in as tightly as possible, which took a good 15 to 30 minutes to do properly. There was great medical attention there, and the Red Cross was there. Even when I was on the wing of that plane in the water, the Red Cross was there helping however they could. Once I got out of the water that last time, they got blankets on me and tried to dry me off.

As I was on that backboard, my pain got worse and worse. I remember that as I laid there, Ed Koch came by, who was the mayor of New York at the time. He put his hand on my shoulder and said, "Sonny, you're going to be fine. We've got the best doctors in the world in New York. They're going to take good care of you." I said, "Thank you Mr. Mayor," and he seemed surprised that I knew who he was. But honestly, who wouldn't know Mayor Koch at that time? The medical team came over and said, "We're going to need a couple of guys to get Mr. Panko in the ambulance." Mayor Koch goes, "We're gonna need more than a couple guys to lift Joe up!" The people around kind of laughed, and as they got some guys to load me into the ambulance, I said, "Mayor Koch, stick with your day job, please." We all laughed about that.

I told them I wanted Jerry to join me in the ambulance, and I'm sure we hit every pothole in New York on the way to the hospital, with the pain getting worse and worse at every bump. They wouldn't administer any painkillers until they found out what was wrong with me. We arrived at the hospital and evidently there were photographers there from television stations. My friend Dr. Fred, a Stanford grad, saw that ambulance footage of me on TV the next morning.

With that, they brought me into the emergency room in Queens Hospital. They immediately put in three IVs for fluids to treat my shock. Then they asked if they could cut off my clothes to attend to me. All of a sudden, three people cut off my clothes at the same time – my left arm, my right arm, and my pant legs. They then discovered that I had this white powder coming out of my vest and they panicked a bit, because they thought it was cocaine or some other illegal substance. I laughed and said, "No. My boss Jerry always likes Equal in his iced tea, and nobody ever has it. So, I always carry it for him." They dug into my vest a little farther, saw the Equal packages and realized I was telling the truth.

The next thing I know, I'm literally naked in New York and the doctors are attending to me. I went to X-ray, which was difficult for me because of the pain. Once they looked at the X-rays and determined the extent of the damage, they administered pain medicine.

I left that particular X-ray room after about an hour to learn that I had severe back damage in my lower discs that was going to cause me a significant amount of problems. I could still move and walk slowly with help or in a wheelchair, but the pain would be extensive for quite a long time.

I was sent back in the emergency room at about 5:00 a.m., when in walked two people wearing suits. There was a gentleman wearing a gray suit with a red tie and a young lady with him in a business suit. They walked over to Jerry and said, "Mr. Holmes, I'm Mr. Andersen and this is Mrs. Jones from IBM." At 5:00 in the morning, IBM was there to help us.

They asked how we were, and we told them what we knew, and they asked what they could do to help us. They talked to Jerry first and helped him with his needs. Then Mrs. Jones said, "Joe, what can I do for you? I said, "Well, I don't have any clothes. I'm naked in New York. See?" I knew I had two sheets on me. So, I grabbed the top sheet and flipped it away. She made an "Oh" sound as if to say you really don't need to show me that you're naked in New York, stupid. She said, "What does that mean?" I replied that I needed everything. So, she got a pad out, and I gave her my sizes for everything from shoes and a shirt to socks, a sweater and a jacket.

After that, they checked us into the hospital. We were both in the same room and we were finally getting something to eat. Or at least Jerry did. They fed Jerry and gave me soup and Jell-O, because I was

THE PLANE CRASH

on a liquids-only diet because of my shock. I was my usual sarcastic self at that point, so I said, "Thanks a lot! Jerry's got chicken. Jerry's got vegetables. Jerry has dessert. Jerry has iced tea. I get Jell-O-and soup."

As we were getting attended to, two people suddenly walked into the room. It was my Uncle Tom Panko, who was retired, and his son Robert, who was a police officer. Robert's boss had seen the footage and told him that his cousin had been in a plane crash. He told him to take a squad car and go see me in the hospital. I hadn't seen my uncle in quite some time, so it was wonderful to see him. They were there for about 15 minutes, when the nurses tried to hustle them out. I asked for a few more minutes, since I hadn't seen him for years, and they gave us a little more time. That was a great mental uplift that someone from my family whom I cared and loved dearly was actually there. It's not that I didn't care about Jerry, but he didn't care about me, so why should I care about him? I'm obviously kidding. I care about Jerry. I love the man for what he's done for both the business and certainly for me personally.

After they left, I felt pretty nasty after being in the slime and whatever they considered water in the East River. I understand that's where the mafia buries people after they dismember them. I always joke that when I finally got my wallet back, there was a finger in it. I guess I watched too many crime shows. So, with that, after they brought me something that passed for food, I decided to try and shower. I got up and all I had around my neck was the collar of the T-shirt. That was the only thing they didn't cut off. That's all I had. No socks, no pants, no underwear, no shirt. I could hardly walk to the shower, and as I slowly walked in front of Jerry, he says, "You know, I've done a lot of things in my life, but now I'm stuck seeing you naked." I said, "I guess it could be worse." He said, "I don't know how." I showered, but not for very long as I could hardly stand.

The nurse came into the room and said that we had a phone call from the chairman of IBM. Jerry took the call. He assured the chairman that we were both fine. I was trying desperately to talk to him, but Jerry wouldn't let me. Again, I'm still in shock and on massive painkillers. I'd been very sarcastic and humorous in this whole episode, both through the evening and that morning, so Jerry was probably pretty wise in not allowing me to get on the phone.

The reason I wanted to talk to the chairman so desperately is that I was responsible for headcount in our division, which was about 12,000 people at the time. It was very important from a business standpoint that we kept track of headcount. We would receive an objective of a certain number, and we had to make sure that we didn't go over that number. Of course, people would come and go, they would get sick, they would go on leave, or they would retire. We replaced them. Sometimes we replaced too many and we were juggling headcount. At the time of the crash, we were 155 people over. The following up and accounting for the headcount is an internal business accounting operation. It has nothing to do with the performance of the corporation. But the President gives you this bogey on headcount, and it's up to us to manage it. Even though he gave us the objective to meet every year, you could get it relieved by the chairman. So, I reasoned that if I talked to the chairman, and I'm 155 headcount over, I could get it relieved. So, I'm in the background of this call between Jerry and the CEO saying that I wanted to talk to him about headcount. Jerry wisely understands that I'm just gutsy enough to ask him for relief at that point in time because (A.) I'm a good employee, (B.) I'm a third generation IBMer, (C.) I was in New York working on a very special product, and (D.) I survived the plane crash, so therefore, (E.) Give me relief. Fortunately or unfortunately, Jerry wouldn't allow me to talk to him. So, with that, I'm still laying here naked, and they brought Jerry more food and they brought me some more Jell-O. So, I'm thinking, this is just great.

All this time, I couldn't really see very well, because my glasses were lost in the crash. They packed me down to the hospital lab where they made me a pair of glasses. They didn't do too well from a prescription standpoint, but it was better than a white cane with a red tip. I got back to the room only to find that the lady with the suit, Mrs. Jones, was back. She had a valise and a briefcase with her, and she pulled out shoes, and socks, and underwear, and a t-shirt and shirt, and a sweater and a jacket. All the things that I needed. There was a toothbrush, and a razor and all the things that I didn't even realize that I needed that I had lost in the water. As I recall, that was about 11:30 a.m.

So, in the span of 12 hours, I'd survived the crash, been in the East River, been to the hospital, had numerous medical procedures, and now I'm getting this help from the great IBM Corporation through Mrs. Jones, only to find out that Hurricane Hugo is about to come through the South and leave a path of devastation through my home in Charlotte, North Carolina.

Sharing is Caring

There were many gifts I was privileged to give to children in hospitals over the years that I hope brightened their days, but perhaps the one that has made me smile the most over the years since was a baby bassinet that I bought from Eckerd Drugstore.

I went to a local hospital with about 6 or 8 gifts to hand out that day, and my first stop was in the room of a little girl who was about 3 years old. I gave her the bassinet that was made for a baby doll, and she asked if it was for her. I answered that yes, it was indeed for her, but in return, she had to promise me that she was going to get better. She enthusiastically responded that she would. With that, I left and went to the next room to share the next gift with another child.

I repeated that process in the next several rooms, but at some point, I happened to look back down the hall and saw that same three-year-old girl happily pushing her baby bassinet from room to room, filling it with each of the toys that I had given to other children.

Needless to say, we had another conversation in which I explained that only the baby bassinet was for her, and that these other toys were meant for other children. After a little encouragement, she got the message and took the gifts back to their rightful owners, making every recipient happy all over again.

The vision of her walking down the hospital hallway with a baby bassinet overflowing with other children's gifts is a memory that I still look back on as being one of the cutest I've experienced.

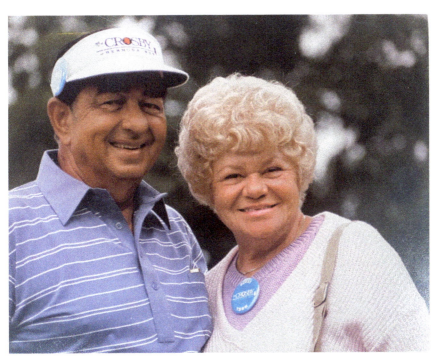

My parents, Olga and Joe Panko at Crosby in North Carolina.

CHAPTER 3

Birth of a Salesman and Childhood Traumas

Throughout my experiences in rehab and beyond, I learned that trauma isn't confined to those major moments in life – the plane crashes, the hurricanes, military combat and the like. There are many things that impact us on a deep psychological level and might not manifest themselves until later in life. For lack of a better analogy, traumas pile up over time, adding layers of complexity that further shape the experiences we have later in life. Oftentimes, we are thankfully unable to recall those that happened very early in life, and as such, we don't really remember how traumatic they were. Once we hit an age that we can remember, however, whether that's two or four or six, they do start to leave an impression that we recall. We might never recognize or identify these singular instances as trauma – they might seem minor to someone else, but they weren't to our tender psyches at the time. As adults we can look back on these moments that shaped us, formed our outlooks and molded our responses to how we process the experiences we encounter later in life.

One of those traumatic experiences literally hit when I was growing up in Binghamton, New York. I was in an apartment with my mother when Hurricane Hazel came through the area. It is very rare for a hurricane to come off the coast that far inland and hit Binghamton. I recall mom and I were in our apartment as the winds got extremely heavy. The scary part for me was that my dad was out building a new home in Endicott, so his reassuring presence wasn't there at the time. We experienced quite a bit of damage and dealt with power outages for some period of time afterward. Even at this age of 73, I can still vividly recall the sound of the wind and the rain tearing at our apartment building as well as witnessing the damage after the fact. Perhaps that was one of the reasons why coming home from a plane crash to Hurricane Hugo in Charlotte hit me so hard.

One interesting incident that happened in Binghamton encouraged my parents to build a new home. I was about four years old, or maybe even five, and I was still sleeping in a crib. It was a big crib, and it was stuck in the corner of this apartment. That was the only thing that would fit there, so they simply couldn't get a bigger bed for me. My mom overheard a conversation between myself and a young boy from a poor family who lived next door. He was in our apartment one day, and his very low voice for his age asked me in astonishment, "Hey, are you still sleeping in a crib? Oh my god." My mother overheard that, realized that it was time for us to get a bigger place, and encouraged my dad to build a new house.

My mom was a beautician at the time. She had gone through a beauty school and gotten a degree in that regard. Our apartment had a spot for her to have her business inside the adjacent apartment, so that had worked out well for her. An interesting thing about mom's career is that she had worked a variety of jobs and worked for IBM in the 1940s. Unfortunately, when she met and married dad, she lost her job. IBM had a policy at that time that married women could not work there. They were trying to give jobs to the men who were coming back from the war.

Mom took it in stride. Her beauty business flourished because of her abilities and talents, her personality, and her knowledge. The new house truly had all the comforts of a new home, and I had my own room, which finally got me out of the crib.

Mom's business, however, was still with us. They designed the house so that as they walked in the front door of our home, clients could walk right down the stairs to the beauty shop in the basement. I don't have a lot of memories about that basement, other than I was always getting reprimanded by my father because my toys were messed up. The reason why my toys got messed up was because they were in the back part of the basement, where the ladies would bring their children. While the moms were getting their hair done, my mom would send their kids back to play with my toys. When it was time for their mothers to leave, they'd go home, and they would leave my toys a mess. There was always a traumatic discussion with my father about why my toys were all over the place. I would protest that "I don't mess them up. I want to keep them in order. But while I'm trying to keep them neat, mom keeps sending these children back here who keep messing them up." That was an interesting part of the new house.

Now my parents drilled into me that it was important for me to be safe on that front staircase. I do remember one morning going downstairs to see my father. Evidently, I wasn't paying attention, and I fell down the stairs. I bounced to the left and to the right, back to the left and then the right. I don't know whether I had a concussion or not, but it was pretty bad. It did afford me a day off from school.

The new house was great in that it gave us a chance to have a beautiful spot for a Christmas tree, and Christmas was always very special. At that age, five or six, I still knew that Santa Claus was coming. This one particular year, Santa Claus came, and I received four beautiful toys, but my mother had 40 packages. I said, "That's not fair. How can I have just four items?" I remember crying and being upset about that. Mom and dad explained to me that Santa Claus has a lot of children to give gifts to, and the gifts for mother were from all her customers. She'd get a sweater or a scarf or perfume from a happy client. Santa Claus did in fact leave me four great presents, they reminded me. So, they conned me into that discussion, and it seemed like I was okay with that. I loved mother dearly and it was great that she got presents from her clients, even if I was initially jealous.

I guess normal kids get bikes at six, seven or eight, but for some reason, either I wasn't normal, or my parents thought it would be more interesting to get me a scooter that had a seat on it. So, I'd clump around the streets of our neighborhood with the scooter while everybody else was riding a bicycle. You ride a scooter with one foot on it and the other foot on the ground, pushing it. So, when I got tired of pushing or I wanted to rest, there was a seat on a scooter. I'm not sure what happened to the scooter, but I'm not really sure why the heck my parents bought me a scooter versus a bike. They never really confessed to that. But as I was growing up, I wondered why do I have this darn scooter when all my friends have bikes? That kind of traumatized me into thinking that either I was different, or I was better than everybody else, so I had a scooter. I'm not sure which way of thinking won in my impressionable mind.

When your parents say, "Don't do this and don't do that," we often do just that, which led to one traumatic incident. My dad and my Uncle Walter were building a home for my Uncle Ted. The three of them were roofing this house and they put me in the corner of the unfinished living room where there was a bunch of wood. They pulled out a few planks for me to pound with nails and said, "No matter what, don't go into pile of wood." What they gave me was flooring oak so tough that the nails I was hammering wouldn't pound into it. I remember thinking this is not very much fun, the nails bend as soon as I hit them, so I'm going to find some other wood. I went into the forbidden woodpile, and I almost immediately stepped on a nail.

The nail went right through my foot. I didn't scream until I pulled the nail out and saw blood. I screamed and I screamed until my dad and my uncle climbed off the roof and asked what happened. I said, "I stepped on a nail." They said, "We told you not to go back there." I said, "I know dad, but I did, and the pain is terrible." So, they rushed me to a doctor for a tetanus shot.

Another doctor experience I don't fondly remember was when my right pinky fingernail got infected somehow. As it got worse, my mom told my dad that he had better take me to the doctor. I'm 73 and I still remember how bad this thing hurt. I went to see the doctor, whose name I can't recall, and he froze my finger so he could pull the fingernail out. Well, my finger hurt enough as it was without him freezing it. When he tore the fingernail out, I started screaming, "Daddy, he's hurting me. Hit him dad, he's hurting me." The pain subsided pretty quickly after the nail was out. They wrapped it up and treated it for infection. I do remember, even at 73 years old, asking the doctor if he had another way out of his office. He said, "Why?" I said, "I don't want to walk in front of the people out there who heard me scream." He replied, "They didn't hear you. We have very thick walls. And so, we went out through the front door, but I do recall people looking at me and they were probably thinking, "That poor kid, they really, really hurt him." I guess, you could say that traumatic experience stayed with me, even though it happened well over 60 years ago.

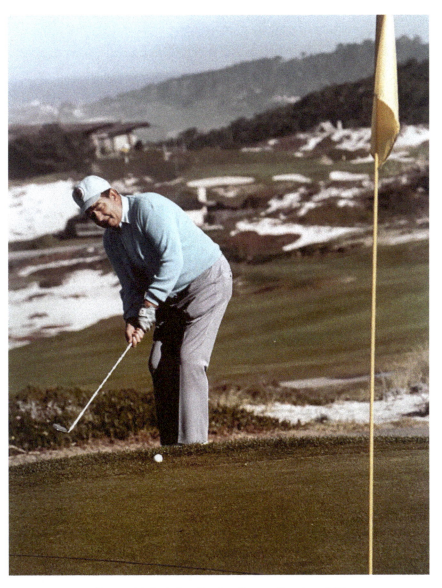

Dear old dad, Joe Panko, Sr., at Spyglass Hill.

As a young man, I had the opportunity to learn how to play chess, checkers, ping pong, golf, pool and billiards at the IBM Country Club Jr. Room. IBM at the time had a country club in many of its locations, and the IBM Country Club at Endicott was flourishing. It was very active in a lot of areas. I don't recall much about bowling there, maybe just once or twice. They had a golf course that was designed by Robert Trent Jones, who was at that time and still is, one of the finest golf course designers in the country. The Interesting thing about watching your parents do things as a young person is that you kind of pick up from them. So, my parents wanted me to learn how to play golf. They bought me a small putter in the pro shop there. I watched my dad putt on the practice putting green before he went off to play. He used to putt different friends of his for nickels. Sometimes he won a dime or a quarter or lost a dime or a quarter, and then they'd go out to play.

I was seven years old at the time. I'd be left at the country club by myself with supervision in the junior room or in the lunchroom. Dad would give me a quarter every day to buy a soft drink or something in the lunchroom. That was certainly a good experience. However, since dad putted for nickels, I started doing it. If you spend hours on a putting green, you know all the breaks and master its nuances. So, I began putting for nickels against random people. I became very proficient and therefore, in my mind, very wealthy. One afternoon, I was done putting and went into the cafeteria. I had maybe $1 to my name and I went in and got a hamburger, French fries, and a milkshake. My dad came in after the ninth hole to get something for himself, and he saw me in there eating this substantial meal. He asked how I got the money for it. I replied that I won it on the putting green, putting for nickels. He said, "You can't be doing that. That's not right." I said, "Well, you do it daddy, so what's different if I do it." He didn't really answer that question but said "You can't be putting for nickels and taking money from all these people." I said, "They don't seem to mind. They think it's kind of funny that a young man can putt so well." He was undeterred and told me to stop doing it. Well, of course, I didn't stop.

One afternoon I putted against a man, and I won 10 holes in a row. The man reached into his pocket, and he didn't have any money. He said, "I don't have any change. but I know and work with your father. I'll give him the money at work." I said, "Okay, mister, that's fine with me." That happened over the weekend.

The next Monday, my dad gets called into the general manager's office at IBM. He's really nervous wondering whether he did something wrong or if he was going to get fired. Dad walked in and the General Manager said, "Good morning, Joe. How are you?" Dad shook the gentleman's hand. The GM said, "Here," and he handed dad two quarters. Dad asked, "What's this?" The GM says, "It's 50 cents." My dad asked, "For what?" The GM said, "Your son beat me out of 50 cents on the putting green." Dad was embarrassed and said, "I told him to stop doing that!" The GM replied, "Let me tell you, your son is one heck of a putter. He beat me 10 holes in a row. After he beat me that bad, I had to quit. I didn't have any change with me, so there's the 50 cents for your son." When daddy got home with my 50 cents, he gave me the money, but I got another lecture about not putting for nickels, although honestly, I still went on to do that from time to time.

In the early years and even more so as I grew up, I always wanted to make things. Unfortunately, I sometimes had the opportunity to make things using incorrect materials. One great example is that my folks got me a set of Lincoln Logs to build things, which were usually used to build cabins and forts and a variety of structures. I had fun doing that. But in those days, children around me were flying kites in the summer, and I didn't have a kite. I figured I could make one using the roofing sticks in the Lincoln Logs. I put those together, taped them as best I could, put newspaper around and taped the whole thing together. As it worked out, I had a beautiful kite. The bad news is that the kite weighed 5 pounds. I tried to get it to fly. It actually flew as long as I was running with it, but there was no amount of wind that could lift that heavy kite. My mom happened to see this spectacle, and she encouraged my dad to buy me a kite.

I now had a very big opportunity to fly a kite with my friends. That's the good news. The bad news is I got this material from my dentist that seemed akin to dental floss. I had this big ball of kite string that was a dental floss type of material. Other children's kite strings were breaking from time to time, but mine was sturdy. The trauma begins when one day when I had the kite as far up as it had ever been, way across the street and way above the trees. The wind changed, and the kite got stuck in the tree. My kite string broke, and I lost my only kite. So that raises another bit of trauma as a young man.

Probably the most traumatic childhood experience I had started when I was an 8-year-old playing Little League baseball. I was proud of my glove. I actually got my first glove at Dick's Sporting Goods, which was started in Binghamton, New York. As you know today, Dick's Sporting Goods is a very popular and proficient sporting goods store providing all kinds of goods and services for families throughout the country. Back in the 1950's, Dick's was a small group of metal buildings. I did pretty well in Little League and was proud of my uniform with the name of our team on the back of it.

My dad got an opportunity to transfer in his job. He was shot up in World War II pretty badly, and fortunately the good Lord and a good doctor saved his legs and saved his life. However, the cold New York winters were bothering his legs. He was in a lot of pain, so he got the idea to move to Arizona. The thought process was that he was going to get a job with IBM in Arizona, and we would live happily ever after there.

As we were leaving town, the most traumatic thing for me as a 9-year-old was taking my uniform on a hanger back to my Little League manager's house. I didn't want to leave. I was leaving all my friends. I was leaving my school. I didn't know what was going to happen.

But my parents said, we have to leave. So here we are outside Mr. Swanson's house, walking up his walkway, ringing the doorbell and handing him my uniform. Mr. Swanson said, "Good luck Joe, you'll do great." Taking my uniform back to my manager was a traumatic experience for my 9-year-old self.

In the process of moving cross country from Endicott, New York, to Arizona, we went through a variety of states. I remember collecting pennants for various things. They might have been state pennants, or one for a particular National Monument like Mount Rushmore. From time to time, I might see a toy that I liked. In New Mexico, I recall that I wanted to buy a particular toy. I had a few dollars in my wallet evidently from my own allowance or from putting for nickels. My dad said, "No, save your money. You don't need it. You can buy something when you get to Arizona."

It was after that that I realized I lost my wallet. We looked here and there but couldn't find it. I said, "See, Dad, if I bought that toy, I would have had that toy now, and I lost my wallet. What am I going to do?" Dad said, "You will earn more money in the future, so don't worry about it." For some reason, my mother must have told people along our route that the hotel we would be staying in was the Arizona Ranch House Inn. A couple of days after checking in there, we got mail. It was strange that we'd get mail, because not very many people knew we were there. It was a small package. We opened that package and inside was my wallet. So, my traumatic experience of losing my wallet turned out to be a lesson in both good fortune, and good friendship. Getting my wallet back along with my mother's insights on helping others played a very important role in my life, and my fascination with toys would certainly play a positive role in how I now help others deal with trauma.

Things went off kilter a bit when we arrived in Arizona. When my dad interviewed at the IBM facility there, they didn't have a position that pertained to what he was trying to achieve in his career. His skills were in manufacturing, whereas theirs were in marketing. They encouraged him to go to San Jose, California, instead. So as dad learned that the type of work he was looking for would only be available in San Jose, he came to the hotel one day and said, "Come on Joe, get out of the pool. We're leaving. We're going to California because they don't have the right kind of work for me." I replied, "That's fine with me. I got my wallet. I got my money. They got swimming pools in San Jose. Let's go."

So, mom, dad and my 9-year-old self moved into the DeDaro Arms apartment for a short period of time until my folks found a place to buy a house. Fortunately, in those days, they had a home show in the area where we were looking. You could come and compare four or five different builders, see their particular houses and the quality of their workmanship, etc. My folks bought a home in an area called Willow Glen that was two streets and two blocks long. This four-square block area was surrounded by cherry orchards, and it was really a great place to grow up. As time went on, more and more homes got built around us, and today it's pretty much wall-to-wall homes. At the time, it was much quieter.

We moved in next to a couple of families, one of which happened to be Leo and Sandy Righetti. The Righetti family had two boys. I was going to be 10 in September; their son Dave was going to be 2 in November and Steve would have been 3 in October. I thought these kids were babies compared to me at the ripe old age of 10. However, when I got to be 15 or 16, I was asked to babysit the young fellows, which was a lot of fun. As I understand it, the Righetti family had a traumatic experience with another babysitter. The other babysitter got into the family's liquor cabinet and was totally inebriated, to the point that they came home to find the babysitter drunk on the couch.

So, I got the job. As I learned, Leo Righetti played professional and semi-pro baseball for a variety of teams. He really didn't like to go back to watch baseball games. Since he knew a lot of coaches and players for a variety of teams, he'd call and get free tickets. I would then take the Righetti brothers to various games in San Francisco in Candlestick Park or in Oakland at the Oakland Coliseum. That was always quite fun.

Flashing back a few years to when we were just moving into our home in Willow Glen. I was going to be 10 years old on September 5, going into the fifth grade, so my parents were faced with the question of where I was going to go to school. The closest was a public school that was a few blocks away, while St. Christopher's Elementary school was maybe a mile away or so. My mom and dad wanted me to go to Catholic school as I did in New York, where I attended Saint Joseph's. So, on the first day of school, I lined up to go into class in what they told me was the fifth-grade line, only to realize that I was in sixth grade instead. After realizing my name wasn't on the roll, they sent me over to the fifth-grade class next door. So, they call the roll from fifth grade - Sarah, Sally, Jimmy and Stevie and whoever, but little Joey's name never got called. So here I am on the first day of school, and I'm already sitting in the principal's office, being asked why they don't have my name on their list. I said, "I was told that I was in this school, and I reported today, and here I am." As it worked out, my mother had been told that there was no room for me in the school; that they were at capacity. However, my mom didn't take no for an answer. She bought me the whole uniform - pants, shirt, sweater, socks, and whatever else we wore back then. The principal, Sister Mary Grace called Father Healy and said "Father Healy, I have this young man Joe Panko here to go into fifth grade, and we don't have him on the list. What are we going to do Father?" Father replied, "We told Mrs. Panko that we were full and that we didn't have room for him." Sister Mary Grace said, "Well, Father he's got the full uniform pants, shirt, sweater, and he's quite a handsome young man. What can we do?" Father Healy said, "Just find another chair, put the chair in the room, and add him to the list." So, for an hour or what felt more like three,

I had this traumatic experience of wondering whether or not I was in school, which was the ideal way to begin middle school in a new city.

The interesting thing about putting for nickels is that it began feeding a pattern. I was always interested in what I could do to make money - whether it was putting for nickels, babysitting in my teenage years, or whatever other ideas I had. But in grammar school, in about the sixth or seventh grade, my career as a salesman was born. I noticed that the school was selling 25 sheets of paper for 10 cents. I saw the same paper at Jolly 5 & 10 for $1 in a 500-sheet ream. I bought the 500 sheets for $1, repackaged the paper, and sold 50 sheets for 10 cents. If I had an opportunity, I looked through the trash cans and found the wrappings of the school's paper so I could use that. As my business flourished and the school's paper business dried up, I got called into the principal's office.

Sister Mary Grace said, "We think you're stealing our paper." That was a difficult concept for me to understand. I replied that I was most definitely not stealing their paper. Sister Mary Grace asked how I could be selling paper with the same wrapping that the school used. I honestly replied, "I am stealing the wrappings out of the wastepaper baskets as people throw them away. I'm using them to package more paper than you provide for 10 cents, and with that, I'm still making a profit. Sister Mary Grace said, "You can't do that. I don't think you're stealing based on what you told me, but you can't do that any longer." I asked, "Why not?" She said, "Because we sell paper as a convenience, and we make money on that paper for school. So, you're out of business." What could an elementary school child do except to say, "Okay."

Then I noticed that Jolly 5 & 10 sold pencils. The school was selling pencils for a nickel each. I bought the same pencils by the dozen at Jolly 5 & 10, and I could sell three pencils for 10 cents. I was selling pencils left and right. Needless to say, the pencils that the school was selling were not selling anymore. After a couple of months, I got called into Sister Mary Grace's office again. "I hear that you're selling pencils," she said. I said, "Yes, ma'am." She said, "Where are you getting them from?" I said, "I get them from the Jolly 5 & 10. I sell the same pencils that you sell for a nickel, but 3 for a dime." It was the same conversation. She said, "We're selling pencils to benefit the school and as a convenience to the children. So therefore, you're out of business." I said "Not again. I was out of business for paper and now I'm out of business for pencils. What am I going to do?" She said, "Go study hard."

At that time, yo-yos became very popular. Kids were playing with all different kinds of yo-yos. They were different colors, some were made of wood, some were made of plastic, and some of them even lit up. Because the strings often broke, yo-yo strings were in demand and were selling in packages of three for a nickel. I got the notion to sell yo-yo strings, but I would buy kite string. I would measure it out on the floor of my house. I would wax it with wax, and the resulting yo-yo strings were sold in sets of five for a nickel. To keep them together, I would use the rubber bands that came with my braces.

As springtime came and more and more kids were using yo-yos string, Sister Mary Grace caught me in the schoolyard, doing a transaction. So, I said, "Good afternoon sister." She said "Joe, how's business?" I said, "Very good, thanks, but don't tell me you're in the yo-yo string business and you're gonna shut me down." She laughed and said, "No, Joe, you can sell all the yo-yo strings you want." So, I finally found my own niche without getting traumatized by upsetting the school.

I shared these stories and a few others that I'll relate later in the book because I think that these are probably similar to what many children go through. At the time, our parents and adults in our lives might not believe that these moments leave a lasting impression, but they do. On a deep level, they shape how we process the events that happen to us later in life.

On the Wings of Love

I believe that sharing gifts and toys with children in hospitals has made a tremendous difference in my recovery, in bringing joy to them and their families, and in some very unexpected places. One of these is within the organizations that have helped me supply the giveaways.

One year, I ran across some small doves that I thought would make wonderful Christmas gifts for children in hospitals during the holiday season. I reached out to the gentleman who owned the company and proceeded to work my normal magic on getting the pieces at a discount. I knew he had way more in stock than he was going to sell, so I proceeded to negotiate the price down from the $5 or so they were to $1 each. At one point, I recall him rather sullenly asking, "What are you going to do with 450 toy doves anyway?" I replied that I was going to give them to sick and dying children in the hospital. I planned on decorating a tree with them and then putting several baskets on the floor around the tree so that kids who were too sick to reach up and pull one off would still be able to get them. He pretty brusquely gave them to me for free at the point. In return, I promised to have the kids send him thank yous. Several weeks later, he called me and said "You need to stop having these kids write to me. I'm reading all these thank yous and tearing up with everyone."

That company owner never planned on impacting the lives of 450 children, but he most certainly did, and I was proud to be able to help him do so.

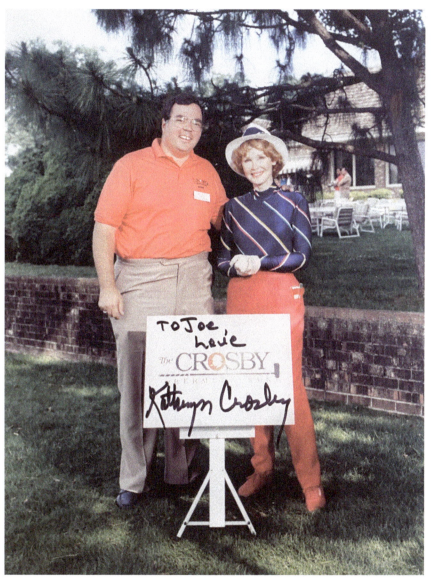

Me with Kathryn Crosby in North Carolina

CHAPTER 4

The Believers Club

Over the years, I've been blessed to have had the opportunity to meet hundreds of interesting people from a variety of walks of life, from entertainment and sports to politics and medicine. I get my personality from my mom. My dad was often embarrassed by her aggressiveness, as she would go to great lengths to meet famous people. That certainly rubbed off on me. I sometimes embarrass my wife with the lengths I'll go to in order to meet certain people. Generally, however, after we meet the person, she's very glad to have taken part in the experience.

The first famous person I ever met was a noted baseball player back in the 1950s. He was a baseman named Johnny Logan from Endicott, New York. I met him when my parents took my 7-year-old self to a wedding in which Johnny was the best man. As a wide-eyed child, I met the shortstop for the Milwaukee Braves in 1956, and in 1957, the Braves went on to win the World Series.

In the early 1960s, my parents took me out of school for a few days because they thought I would enjoy going to the Tournament Champions golf tournament at the Desert Inn Golf Club and Resort in Las Vegas, where all past champions would congregate at the Del Webb Desert Inn. I got a chance to meet quite a few golfers at the time, but since

I was 13, I don't really remember who. A decade or so later, when I worked for the Crosby family in the 1970s, I certainly met folks I recalled meeting back at that first golf tournament experience.

One interesting thing about Las Vegas at the time was that across from the Desert Inn was a small western town designed for children. Parents would drop children off to play games or maybe enjoy a few small rides and the like. The town was made up of small buildings: the general store, the jail, the bank, the hotel, and a variety of others. My parents dropped me there and said they would pick me up at 4 p.m. At the time, I loved playing pinball. I found this little building that had three or four pinball machines. I had a few dollars, so I put in a quarter, and I ended up winning and winning and winning. After two hours of playing this one particular machine, I looked at my watch and saw it was 4 p.m. I had a dilemma. I had 20 free games available to play, but it was important that I met my folks at the gate at 4 p.m., because we were going to go to dinner and a show at the Riviera that evening.

The need to please my parents won out. I left the pinball machine and stepped out on the porch of the small building. There was a tall gentleman standing there and he said, "How you doing little boy?" I said, "Fine sir. What's going on?" He said, "They're filming a movie here." I said, "Really? Who's in it?" He said, "Anne Margaret and Elvis Presley." I looked up at him and said, "Well, isn't that you?" He said, "Yeah."

Well as soon as Elvis said, "Nice to meet you," this guard screamed at me like I had just robbed a bank. He was screaming, "You're not supposed to be here. What are you doing here?" I replied, "I've been in this building for the last two and a half hours, and I'm supposed to meet my parents at 4 p.m. at the front gate." He screamed at me, "Come on. I'll take you to the gate." Elvis looked at me and said, "You take care little boy." I said, "Okay, good luck." He said, "Thank you. Same to you." That was my 30 seconds of history with a great American talent. I later learned that the movie he was filming was *Viva*

Las Vegas. If you watch that movie, there is a 20 second cut of that little Western town, and I think he is actually standing on the porch where I met him.

I really didn't tell my parents about the meeting because I was far more concerned about getting yelled at by the guard. My folks took me back to the hotel, and we got dressed up for the dinner show where we saw the original New York cast of *Flower Drum Song*, and we really enjoyed that. The star of that show was a gentleman by the name of Jack Soo. And lo and behold, after the show was over, we were getting the car, and I had the opportunity to meet Jack Soo. He later played one of the policemen in a sitcom called *Barney Miller*. So, I met those two celebrities along with some golf names at the age of about 13, and I was hooked.

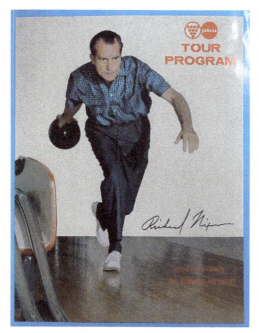

President Nixon personally signed my cover of the Professional Bowlers Tour Program.

My mom and dad bowled quite a bit. My opportunity to play sports was predominantly in the baseball realm, but I bowled on the weekends. The IBM company had intramurals for families, including bowling and softball leagues. The season culminated with the awarding of a large trophy they named after the founder of the company, Thomas Watson. The Watson Trophy Dinner was always something special. As time progressed in the late 1960s, I got better at bowling. My dad purchased a new bowling ball for me.

Unfortunately, it didn't work very well, and he asked me if I was going to give up the sport. As time went on, he got me some lessons from a lady named Betty Patavina, a female professional bowler who taught me quite a few things about my game. Thanks to her and lots of practice, I got better and better. I think I averaged 154 that next year. I bowled extremely well one particular weekend, and I won the First California Junior State Championship. I came in third in doubles with a friend of mine, and I ended up winning the All Events, which was a combination of Team Bowling, Doubles Bowling and Singles Bowling, which is a nine-game block.

As my game improved, I organized the bowling team in my high school and helped organize the bowling league for other area high schools. We traveled once a week to different Bowling Centers, which was a lot of fun. That particular year, I averaged 213 for a short number of games, which ended up being one of, if not the, highest average in the country that year for an amateur bowler. With that achievement came an opportunity to try out for a bowling program organized by the Smallcomb Enterprise Organization. Glen Smallcomb was a young multimillionaire back in the 1960s. He had raised his money from his parents' automobile business and started an organization of Professional Bowlers and women bowlers. In 1967-68, he started an amateur boys' team of 12 to 13 players. Unfortunately, I was not picked the first year, which was very depressing. You talk about traumatic experiences, that particular experience, like the one early on with the bowling ball, motivated me to get better in the game and as a person, which I did in my junior and senior years.

The second time I tried out, I made the team. What was special about making the Smallcomb team that particular year was that we had the opportunity to go to Hawaii for a month. Junior Bowling, along with Pop Warner Football and Little League baseball, went to help the Hawaiian kids get off the beaches and play more sports. That was a terrific opportunity to meet a lot of people in the sport. As it worked out, we bowled 18 exhibitions in 21 days. Glen's business manager,

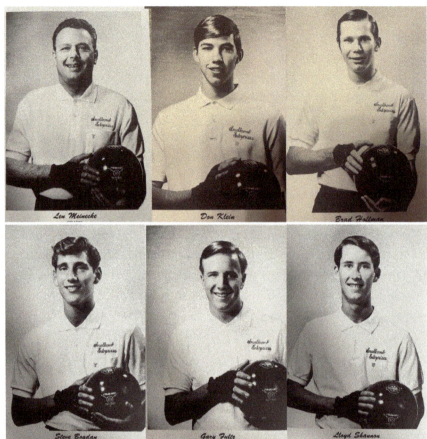

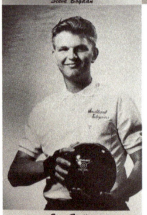

All the members I bowled with on the Smallcomb junior staff.
Mom and dad with bowling great Don Carter.

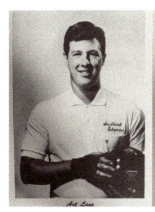
Art Lane

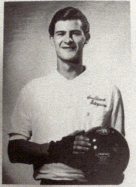
Barry Brady

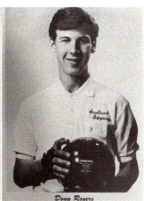
Doug Rogers

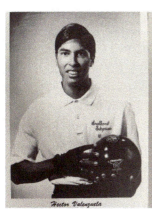
Hector Valenzuela

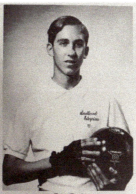
Phil Ruth

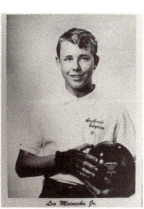
Len Meinecke, Jr.

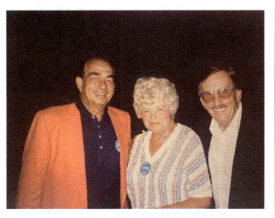

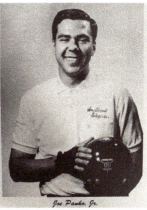
Joe Panko, Jr.

Tim Hoffman, Jr., was extremely instrumental in promoting what we were doing in Hawaii. Each of us got about 500 or so cards with our pictures that we got to autograph for the children we were meeting. So here we are at 15, 16 and 17 years old, signing autographs. Many of the folks I went to Hawaii with are still friends, like Hector Valenzuela, Steve Findley, Phil Ruth, Len Meinecke Jr., and others. We did a lot of advertising for Pan American Airlines, and they sponsored our flights over and back. We were dressed by King Louis bowling apparel, with Hyde bowling shoes and Ebonite bowling balls. This equipment was all brand new, so we got to introduce it into the marketplace, for both adult and junior bowling. We were treated royally for the entire time we were there.

As we went through the week, we faced a variety of conditions. Some of us bowled well and others not so much. Coming from the Bay Area where there was no humidity and flying to Hawaii for the first time, it was very challenging. I don't recall his name, but we met the governor of the state of Hawaii at the time. This opportunity gave me the chance to improve my game and meet a lot of folks. In college, I volunteered to teach my PE professors' bowling classes. That gave them a spare hour or two to do other things. It also gave me the opportunity to learn more about the game, learn how to promote the game, and why it was important to have people participate in the game, even if they only averaged 120 or 140.

I was unable to continue to be a junior bowler because of my age, but through a friend of the family, I was able to secure a bowling sponsor for 10 weeks on the Summer Tour between my junior and senior college years, which was extremely exciting. Because of the Smallcomb Staff, I met some special friends, such as Carmen Salavino, the great Don Carter, and Jim St. John, who later became my neighbor, along with Glenn Allison, Dave Soutar, Skee Foremsky and the like. I was comfortable in the pros, and I thought I would do fine. Even though I was the young pro, I got an opportunity to do the Pro Am in Fresno. I started on the low end of the house, on lanes 3 and 4. I started striking and striking. When I started bowling, the only people following me were an older lady and a guard, but as I got 9 strikes in a row, there were 50 people watching me. Next thing I know, I had 10 strikes in a row and there were 200 people watching me and the whole center stopped bowling to watch. Unfortunately, I didn't strike on the last ball and shot a 299 in the Pro Am. I still remember Carmen Salvino giving me a hard time for stealing his public away. He was such an animator that he would have hundreds of people watching him everywhere he went.

That was the most fun I had on the tour. I didn't bowl very well and didn't get a check week after week after week. I was in a very traumatic state, having to repeatedly call my sponsor Bruce Edwards and tell him I didn't cash. He was happy that I did as well as I did, some weeks coming closer than others. In Houston I bowled terribly. I was in the locker room crying when the Director of the Professional Bowlers Association, Harry Golden, saw me and said, "I know you had a tough time, but how about working the board for me this week?" I said, "That'd be great. Thank you." What that entailed was keeping an ongoing scoreboard for the fans to know how each of the players was progressing. The good news was that it paid $100. When I got the $100 check, I mailed it to my sponsor. That was the sum of money I was able to return to my sponsor that first year.

As I continued to bowl, I met Nelson Burton, Jr. and Dick Weber and developed a lot of friends in the game. I invited Bones Yamasaki and Taro Misato to stay in our home while they bowled the San Jose professional tournament. My parents had a terrific dinner for the Smallcomb staff with Buzz Fazio, Glenn Allison, and Jim St. John. We had a ping pong table as our dining table with a dozen people gathered around it. My dad did a great job with steaks and Italian sausage. My mom made halupkies, which are pigs in a blanket, and Buzz Fazio the Italian man loved those. It worked out Buzz Fazio and Johnny Guenther made the TV finals. So, me and my soon-to-be wife, Susan, sat behind the bowlers on ABC Sports next to Buzz' wife. Bud Palmer was the announcer that day.

As the tournament went on, John Guenther started bowling strikes on national TV - 1, 2, 7, 8, 9, and 10 strikes, all the way to 300. It was a 300 game bowled on national TV. That particular show is still on YouTube. If you search for Johnny Guenther's 300 game, you'll see Susan and me sitting in the audience. I'm wearing a yellow sport coat with a Smallcomb Enterprises staff logo, and you'll watch one of the greatest moments in bowling history.

While bowling allowed me to meet folks from a variety of fields, I always wanted to be a part of golf. My folks took me to the Bing Crosby Golf Tournament as I was growing up. I would walk the fairways and see various celebrities like Phil Harris and James Garner, but I never really met them. One weekend, my parents had an opportunity to meet a family who owned a house at Pebble Beach. A couple of weeks later, my fiancée at the time, Suzi, and I went to Monterey. I said, "Let's stop and see these folks." Well Suzi didn't want to. It was just like my mom and dad all over again, and just like my mom, I won. So, we went to their house and knocked on the door.

I told the woman who answered the door about my mother, and how she had met them at a particular restaurant called Rocky Point. But I had the story wrong. To everything I said, this woman said, "No." Finally, the woman said, "I'll get my husband, maybe he'll remember." This gentleman's name was Charles Kramer. He, too, told me I had my story all wrong, but he invited us in anyway. Even though Mr. Kramer was under the weather, he gave us a tour of the house and a tour of the Beach Club. After two hours, we escaped. During that time, I asked him if he knew how I could become a Crosby Marshal. He said, "I know the guy who runs it. I'm seeing him next week. You send him a note, and we'll see what we can do." Well, I knew the waiting list was very long, so I didn't hold out much hope. A short time later, I got a postcard in the mail that simply said, "Give us your shirt size and your jacket size," and with that I became a Crosby Marshal.

That was extremely exciting in that I got to participate from Monday through Sunday at three courses, Cypress Point, Spyglass Hill, and Pebble Beach. The first day I worked as a marshal at Cypress Point, I was working in the first tee box. There weren't many people out there on that Monday. Frank Thacker was a retired professional who was the starter at Cypress Point that day. This gentleman walked up to him and said, "I would like to play." Frank said. "I'm sorry, I just don't know your name." The gentleman said, "That's quite alright." He took his hat off and said, "I'm Sean Connery."

On Tuesday, I got to follow Nathaniel Crosby and Clint Eastwood. When I walked with them, I was able to take some pictures because my particular job was over for the day. The fun part about meeting all these people over the years is that I've taken thousands of pictures. I've had many of them blown up to 8" x 10", and then the following year, I would bring them back and get the individuals in them to sign them for my collection.

The Wednesday before the tournament. I walked out to the 13th hole. I stopped at 13 because Ken Venturi was there. He was a prominent professional out of San Francisco. He was playing with a young man named Duncan Johnson, and the director and producer of CBS golf, Frank Chirkinian. The 13th green is large, and the flag pin was in the center of the green. Ken put three golf balls down, and he said to Frank, "Watch this. One putt you can hit right, one putt you can hit left, and one putt you can hit straight." He sank all three of those 20' putts. It was really spectacular to see Ken's talent. We walked up the 14th fairway just as it started to sprinkle, and this guy comes out of the woods with an umbrella. He said, "Can I join you?" And lo and behold, it was James Garner. At that time, Jim was extremely popular, not only in movies but in *The Rockford Files* TV show.

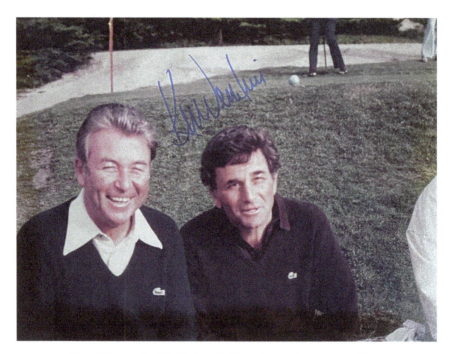

Ken Venturi with Peter Falk, who stole my cookies, at Cypress Point Club in 1976.

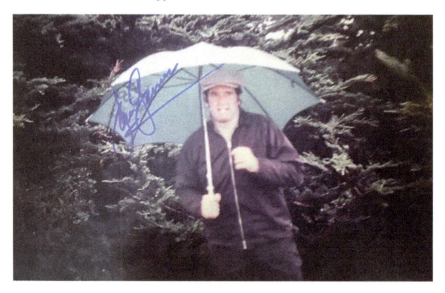

James Garner joining us to play Cypress Point Club.

I was extremely excited to be part of this group walking in. As we finished the 14th and were playing underneath the trees on the 15th, there was an old man sitting on a large stump that's kind of like a bench. It's been there for years. I sat next to him, and I was eating some cookies that Susan had made. The guy says, "What are you eating?" I said, "Cookies." He goes, "What kind?" I said, "They're chocolate chip cookies." He goes, "Oh, where'd you get them?" I said, "My wife, Susan made them for me." He said, "Oh. Are they any good?" I said, "They're delicious." So, you know, obviously, he's trying to get me to ask him if he wants one. I said, "After all those questions, would you like to have one?" He says, "I thought you'd never ask." Everybody in the foursome started laughing. With that I shared a couple of cookies with a gentleman named Peter Falk. He was known for the TV show *Colombo*. He was also in the movie *Robin and The Seven Hoods* with Frank Sinatra and the Rat Pack.

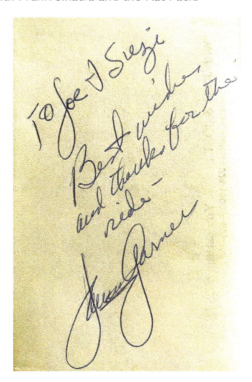

James Garner thanks me for a ride to the lodge at Pebble Beach.

We finished the 18th hole with this group, and most of them went on their way. Since I got there early, my car was parked up front, and I saw James Garner sitting on my car as he was talking with Frank. He was looking for his friends, saying "Where is Sammy? He was supposed to pick me up and take me to the lodge." I said, "I'll be glad to give you a ride, Mr. Garner." He said, "Call me Jim, and where's your car?" I said, "You are sitting on it." He apologized and got in the car. I put the key in the hole and froze for a moment because I was stunned that James Garner is sitting in the front seat of my car. He read my mind. "I know you can't believe I'm sitting here in your darn car. Now let's go." I said, "Yes sir," and I went the way I knew. He said, "You're going the wrong way." I said, "No, this will get you there faster." Sure enough, I got there quicker than he thought. When we got to the back gates, the guard said, "You can't come in this way." I said, "I'm with James Garner." The guy says, "You still can't come in this way." All of a sudden, the caddy gets out of the back of the car and says, "This is James Garner. Don't you know who he is? What do you live in a cave?" Finally, the guard let us in.

As I was parking the car, I said, "I'm going to have to change in the restroom." James Garner asked, "Change for what?" I said, "I'm going to the clambake tonight, which is a party to thank all the volunteers for their work. I have to change my clothes." He asked, "Where are you staying?" I said I'm staying in Monterey." He said, "You don't have to change in the restroom; change in my room." I said, "That'd be great." The next thing I know, I'm in James Garner's suite, changing my clothes to go to the clambake. He asked again, "Where are you staying. I said, "I'm staying at a place in Monterrey. It's clean and it's affordable." After several attempts to get more info out of me, he blurted out, "Where the heck are you staying?" I said, "Jim, I'm staying at Motel Six." He said, "Really. Motel Six," kind of rolling his eyes. So, with that I went to the clambake, and that's what started our relationship over many, many years.

We'd chat every year and I'd see him here and there. About 10 years later, I was done working and I was resting in my room. I'd taken my uniform off and I was just lying there in my skivvies, when a manager knocked on the door. Now, in the early years of Motel Six, they didn't even have phones in the room. If you had to talk to someone, you would call on a payphone outside the lobby or the manager would come to your room if you got a call. Here was the manager saying, "You got a phone call." I said, "Okay, I'll be right there." He said, "Well hurry up." I asked, "Who is it?" I figured maybe it was my parents or there was a problem with them in San Jose. He replied, "It's James Garner." I got dressed quickly, went to the office and said, "Good afternoon." Jim said, "What are you doing?" I said, "I just got back from work, and I was freshening up. I'm watching golf." He said, "There's a party tonight and I want you to join us." I said, "That's great, but how did you know I was here?" He says, "Joe, I'm with a guy who owns Motel Sixes throughout the state of California and other states. He owns more than 50 of them, and you're the only asshole I know who has ever stayed at one."

I ended up getting dressed and going to the party. I met a wide variety of people in show business, such as Phil Harris, Jack Lemmon, Glen Campbell, John Denver, and Sean Connery was there again. It was a lovely evening of mingling amongst the folks talking about the golf tournament.

Opportunities like that came from working the Crosby for many, many years. One of the interesting things that I got to do was I was working at Cypress Point when President Gerald Ford played there. I was alongside of him marshaling on the first hole, along with the Secret Service folks. He was playing with Arnold Palmer that year. About 15 years later, a friend of mine who worked at the *San Jose Mercury News* said, "Joe I'm retiring and when I was cleaning out my office, I found something for you." He handed me a picture of myself working as a marshal on the first green of Cypress Point standing next to the President of the United States.

Years later, I got to meet President Ford when he played the 15th hole at Spyglass Hill. The 15th is a par three. It's the shortest hole on the course but very challenging with water on the right and a green that's shaped almost like Africa. That particular year, Ford was playing with Jack Nicklaus. Unfortunately, the President was known for wild shots. He shanked his tee shot off to the right and hit a lady in her head and cut her head open. It was like the cuts boxers get, there's a lot of blood but it's not really bad, but it was a bad situation. I was attending to her and getting medical folks there. As she was resting on the ground, her husband was going berserk. He was nose to nose with the president yelling, "If you can't play any better, you shouldn't be playing. Look at my wife, she's all bloody. What are you going to do about it?" As he got more and more aggressive, these two Secret Service guys picked him up. He was somewhat of a short man, so his legs were swinging back and forth.

In the meantime, I was coming down the hill and Jack Nicklaus asked me if the President was going to play, meaning whether Jack could take another shot. I knew where Jack was on the green and I yelled, "He said to go ahead and knock it straight in." Jack couldn't hear me. As I got closer to the green, Jack said, "Pardon me, what did you say?" I said, "He said go ahead and play, and knock it straight in, if you get my drift." He kind of nodded at me. The President was coming down the hill as the lady was being attended to and the Secret Service was taking care of her husband, and Jack Nicklaus made a 30' birdie putt. Jack Nicklaus walked by me and said, "Joe, I got your drift." Meaning that I knew the putt was straight in, because I'd been standing there for the last four days watching every shot.

Over the years, I worked the practice tee to help out, picking up ball buckets and giving people information. The next day, the President came to the practice tee with his caddy, and there was a spot for him to hit balls right next to Fuzzy Zoeller. Fuzzy was a character from Indiana who turned out to be a great friend over the years. Fuzzy said, "Mr. President, there's a spot right over here." Gerald Ford put this bag down and he was going to start hitting balls, when Fuzzy says, "Excuse me sir, but just a minute." Fuzzy reached in his golf bag, pulled out a Stanford football helmet, put it on and said "Okay – now go ahead and hit!" He made the paper, and it was a great bit of humor that Ford took well. The President went on and played well in the next few rounds and came back several other times.

I had an opportunity to speak with Gerald Ford numerous other times over the years. One time I was with some IBM friends at the Pebble Beach Lodge. We were about to order some drinks and I went to the restaurant. On the way Gerald Ford walked by me and I said, "Mr. President, can you stop by and see my boys over there by the fireplace." He said, "Joe, I'm doing an interview in another room. I'll stop by and see them after." I went back to my friends and said, "Did you see the President walk by? He's going to come by and see us later." They said, "Yeah, right." I sat down as the beverages came, and sure enough, the President stopped by and said, "How are you folks doing? My friend Joe asked me to stop by after my interview." They were sitting there with their mouths open. It was fun to have that interchange.

The tournament led me to have a good acquaintance with Phil Harris. He was a very close friend of Bing Crosby's. I only met Bing Cosby once before he passed away and I met him while I was working for Glen Smallcomb. Glen would have me go get his car washed, pick up his laundry, do his banking, and pick up some groceries from time to time. I always enjoyed doing that, because his car was a 1966 Rolls Royce. Needless to say, I kept back at least 10 car lengths every time I drove it. Glen also loved chocolate chip cookies made by a famous restaurant called Stickney's in Palo Alto, California.

Stickney's was known for having a great bakery, but once they sold out of something for the day, it was gone. One day, Glen sent me out to get the car washed, and to get him chocolate chip cookies from Stickney's. I was standing behind this older gentleman at Stickney's, and as he ordered, he said, "I'll get those last three chocolate chip cookies." I said, "You can't do that. You can't buy those chocolates chip cookies." He asked, "Why?" I said, "I was supposed to get those for my boss. That's what he wants." He asked, "Well, what's his second favorite?" I said, "Oatmeal raisin." He said, "Give this young man two dozen oatmeal raisin for his boss." The older gentleman turned around and it was Bing Crosby,

I made a valiant attempt to get him to sacrifice those three cookies for my boss. Finally, he asked. "Who's your boss?" I said, "Glen Smallcomb." He said, "Tell Glen I bought the last three chocolate chip cookies." I went back to the office, and handed Glen his laundry, his banking and his change from the cookies, which was the $20 bill he gave me. He asked, "How could you buy cookies and still have $20 left?" I said, "Because an older gentleman in front of me bought the cookies." Glen opened the box and said, "These aren't chocolate chip, these are oatmeal raisin?" I said, "Because he bought the last three chocolate chip cookies." Glen said, "Come on. You couldn't talk him out of it? I know you could have talked him out of it." I said, "No. He was very nice, and he bought the two dozen for you." Finally, Glen said, "Who was it?" I said, "It was Bing Crosby." Glen picks up the phone and dials Mr. Crosby, and before Bing could even answer. He says, "It's Glen. You got the last three chocolate chip cookies! How come you didn't let Joe get the last cookies? I could hear. Mr. Cosby laughing on the phone. The exchange went on for several minutes, and that's how I met Bing Crosby.

As time went on, more and more unique things happened, one of which was I developed a friendship with Peter Jacobsen, a terrific flamboyant young man and player at the time who always played with Jack Lemmon. Jack is a great comedian, who played with Tony Curtis and Walter Matthau in many movies. Now the 15th Hole is a short par three. Jack would always hit the ball to the left, down this hill and off the green. I'd have to go over and move the ropes, move the people and make it secure so Jack could hit a shot. When he did this for the umpteenth year in a row, I walked over to him and said "Jack, every year, year after year, you always hit left. Look at how big this green is. It's only 130 yards, Jack, you can't hit it left." He says, "Joe. Be quiet. Just move the ropes and let me hit my shot." I said, "Okay, but next year please try to get closer to the flag." We laughed. He gave me a wink and he hit his next shot, and sure enough the next year he was over there again.

Over the years, Jack Lemmon never made the cut to play on Sunday. That was the sad, sad tale of Jack's golf game. But I befriended him and got a chance to meet numerous folks who played with him. One year, the Crosby boys stopped at my hole and introduced me to the person they were playing with. He said, "This gentleman Joe Panko has been with us for many years. He's a very loyal Marshal." The name of the person they introduced me to was Donald Trump. That was a few holes before he made a hole in one on the 12th hole at Spyglass. It was a thrill to meet him and at the time I didn't know Donald Trump from Colonel Sanders, but as time went on, we know the story there.

I would experience three holes in one there over the years. One by a gentleman named Richard Gelb, who at the time was the Chairman of the Board of Bristol Myers company. And lo and behold, he hit a wedge or a nine iron and after a few bounces, it went in the hole. Another by a young man named Johnny Miller, Jr. After Johnny hit the ball in the hole, his father hit the ball three feet past the hole, and then it spun back and rimmed the cup, ending two inches from the hole. It would have been a back-to-back, father and son hole in one. The other hole in one was made by a man who is a day older than me. This gentleman is a very famous golfer who won several masters tournaments. He hit the ball, and two bounces later, it went in the hole. That was Tom Watson, and he has been a good friend for years. Because he's a day older than I am, I send him birthday cards, and recently because of my ailments and his losing his wife, he has sent me quite a few handwritten notes.

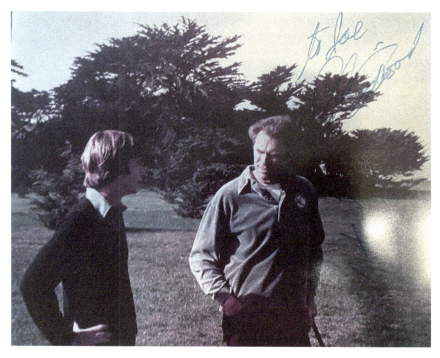

Clint Eastwood made my day when he finally signed this.

The year I marshaled at Cypress Point, I got a terrific picture of Nathaniel Crosby and Clint Eastwood playing there. The next year, I brought that picture and had Nathaniel sign my 8" x 10". I saw Cint Eastwood one morning, and I said, "Clint, I'm Joe Panko and I took this picture at Cypress Point. I'd really appreciate it if you'd sign this picture for me to complete the pair." He said, "I can't do it right now. I'm in a rush." Well, I've learned over the years that if you don't get a signature when you can, you might never have the opportunity to get it again. He was by himself, and he was carrying his own bag. I said, "I'll carry your bag, and you can sign the picture while we walk." He said, "I told you I was late." I said, "Let me just carry the bag and let you complete the pair of signatures." He still hemmed and hawed, so I said, "Clint, why don't you just sign J-E-R-K, and they'll know who it is." He said, "Give me that!" and he signed me a really beautiful Clint Eastwood and said, "I like you." I replied,

"You're a great actor and a big asset to this tournament, so I really appreciate you signing it."

As time went on, I'd see him and he'd always stop and say hi, so we were really good acquaintances. Years later, after the plane crash I'd taken my employee Ed Hatch to Pebble Beach. On one of the practice days, they'd have a shootout for charity. There was Clint Eastwood on the 18th Green, and Ed and I were standing close by. Clint acknowledged me and I asked him to come over, and he nodded his head that he would. There were probably 100 people around Ed and me. As the awards got presented and Clint was done, he walked over, said, "Joe, how you doing after the accident?" I said, "I'm making progress but still not up to par. Would you sign a few things for me?" He looked at me and smiled and said, "Joe, I'll always sign things for you." All these people are going, "He didn't sign anything for us!" One lady made a comment, "Who is this Joe guy. Nobody really knows who Joe is?" That was a fun exchange, which I've had quite a few of with Clint over the years.

As I mentioned earlier, a lot of folks didn't believe my stories when I moved from San Jose to Charlotte and came back to work the golf tournament as a Marshal. After two or three years, word got around the IBM facility that none of my stories were true. So, I stopped telling them. People would ask me how the tournament was when I came back and I'd say, "The weather was good, and there was great golf." People would say, "Why don't you tell us more?" I'd say, "Because you're a bunch of non-believers." A buddy of mine, John Ostrander, who's been a friend for many many years, started a believers and non-believers club.

I would tell a story and people would be excited to hear it and afterward, John would say they are either non-believers or believers and we laughed about that. One particular year, Bob Fritch said "I want to join you so I can be a member of the believer club." We went and stayed at my parents' house. I told him, "Tomorrow we have a breakfast meeting. We'll go to breakfast and then we'll go from there to Pebble Beach." That morning we drove to Hillsboro, California. We drove through the gate of this estate, parked the car, walked up and rang the doorbell. This lady answered the door, gave me a hug, and said it was great to see me. Her name was Kathryn Crosby.

So, we had breakfast at Kathryn Crosby's house. Bing had unfortunately passed away by then. Kathryn moved the tournament from Pebble Beach to Advance, North Carolina, by Winston Salem to raise money for Alzheimer's. There was a disagreement between the Crosby family and the Professional Golfers Association. They wanted to call it the Bing Crosby AT&T national Pro Am. Catherine said, "No. It's Bing's tournament, no other names should be added to it." And with that disagreement she moved the tournament to North Carolina.

I was appointed by Frank Schlage to talk with Kathryn regarding my running the marshals for the first year or two. That was our discussion that morning. That afternoon, Bob Fritch and I checked into the famous Motel Six and went to the Lodge at Pebble Beach. As we were standing in the large lobby, someone walked by and said, "Joe, it's good to see you this year." I said, "This is my friend Bob Fritch." And Bob Fritch with his mouth open, shook the hand of Clint Eastwood. After Kathryn Crosby and Clint Eastwood in the same day, Bob said, "Joe, I'm a believer, I'm a believer."

So, the interaction with folks at IBM only got better over time. I worked in the Executive Briefing Center, which was the place where we brought bank executives and presidents from throughout the world to view our products and sign contracts to install the great IBM banking equipment. I was the manager of international briefings, so I would meet with bank presidents from Spain, Italy, France, the British Isles, Africa, China, Japan, and the like. I would coordinate presentations regarding the technical aspects of the machinery, and perhaps take them to dinner at various places in Charlotte.

One of the most memorable meetings I've had was with the president of the Bank of Spain. He was not very pleased with IBM equipment. His technical people liked it, but for some reason he wasn't pleased with us. I didn't really understand the entire story. I knew who he was, and I knew that his son-in-law was very famous. I also knew that I had a picture of his son-in-law and one of my best friends, Dr. Fred Martinez, in my office. After I gave my presentation and we took a break for some beverages, I said, "Sir, I'd like you to come to my office and see this picture." His interpreter said, "Okay." The president of my division was there and he asked, "What are you doing?" I said, "Just follow me, sir." We came around the corner into my office, which was small and just had a desk and a couple chairs. But the Bank of Spain president walked into my office and saw this 20" by 30" framed photograph, and he started yelling and screaming. "That's my son in law Seve Ballesteros. He's married to my daughter Carmen. He's a great athlete; he's a Masters champion." He kept going on and on, so his attitude toward IBM changed from laissez faire to very positive. The rest of the meeting went well. They signed one of the largest contracts that we had at IBM. My president said, "You took a chance, young man, and you did a great job." He gave me a dinner for two, for me and my wife Susan which was an informal award that they pass on from time to time. John was there and he looked at me and said, "Well, the president of the bank is now a member of the believers club."

There were quite a few fun instances I had with Sean Connery. Pat Saign, a high school friend of mine, and his wife were coming from the Bay Area to Pebble Beach to have dinner with me. I kept getting up and walking to the front desk to see where they were. Jack Lemmon asked what I was doing, and I explained the situation and that my friend was a half hour late. Well, in the interchange before that, I was at the front desk at the lodge waiting for Pat, and there was Sean Connery with his wife along with Bob Hoge and his wife and they were waiting to go to a party. He also asked why I kept coming to the front, and I explained that Pat was running late. He said, "That's not kosher." I said, "You're right. When he shows up, give him a hard time." About 10 minutes later, they were still standing there waiting for their ride when Pat came across the putting green at Pebble Beach. Sean Connery waylaid him and said, "Pat, you're 30 minutes late, that's unreasonable. You now have to pay for all the dinners and drinks and desserts. Pat is smiling because he knows that I put Sean up to it, while Pat's wife is in shock over the whole thing.

Finally, we get downstairs and about 20 minutes later, Jack comes by the table and says "Glad you could show up Pat. People have been waiting around here and they're waiting for this table. You're delaying dinner. You are supposed to eat and then get the hell out of here so somebody else can eat. Instead, you're over here running 30 minutes late."

The opportunity to take pictures of people and get them to sign them the next year opened the door to many of these relationships. I took this picture of Robert Wagner, who was playing with Burt Lancaster that next year. I had stopped Mr. Wagner at the practice tee to sign my picture. He said, "I'll be glad to." Burt Lancaster starts yelling at him. "We're always late. You don't know where the hell you are going here." I said, "Excuse me, where are you playing today?" He said, "Cypress Point." I said, "I'll give you easy directions." So, Robert Wagner signs the picture for me, and I gave them good directions. Burt was skeptical, but I said, "Follow these directions and you'll get there so early that you'll even have time enough to putt." The next day, Burt Lancaster and Robert Wagner played my hole. Burt Lancaster came by me, and I took a few pictures of him. He said, "Young man, I owe you an apology. I was yelling yesterday. You got me there early so I could practice putting and I played well all day long because of that." As he was leaving, he gave me a smile and I said, "Thanks again Jim

Thorpe." He played Jim Thorpe in one of my favorite all time movies, and he gave me a smile and a wink, just like he did in the movie *Field of Dreams*. I still melt every time I see him smile at Kevin Costner and give him a wink in *Field of Dreams* because that's the wink I got in the picture.

Perhaps because of these experiences, I learned from an early age on the importance of spreading joy where and when you can. Many of these celebrities did so simply by signing a picture, teasing a friend, or just taking a moment to talk. In my own life, after the accident, I was to take that lesson about giving time and small gifts and transform it into a positive coping mechanism that would change the way I dealt with trauma, and I hope, make a positive impact on the lives of many others as well.

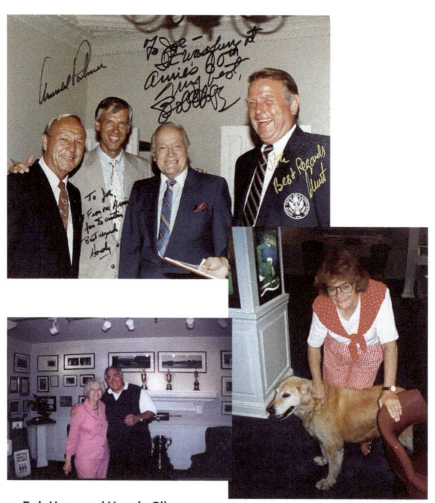

Bob Hope and Howdy Giles celebrating Arnie's 60th birthday. Winnie Palmer with Riley in Latrobe. Debbie, Gina and me in Arnie's Latrobe office.

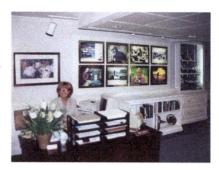

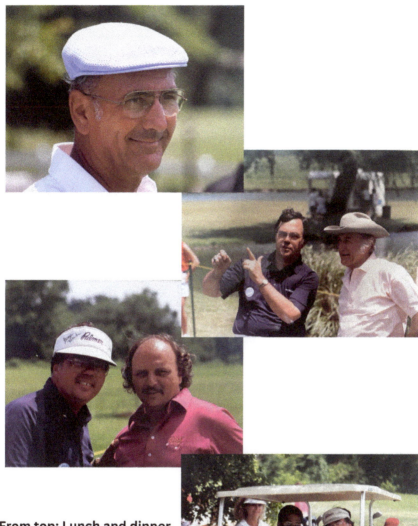

From top: Lunch and dinner fun with Celtic great Bob Cousey. Fishing great Grits Grisham at the Crosby. Crosby regular Dennis Franz. Basketball great "Doctor J."

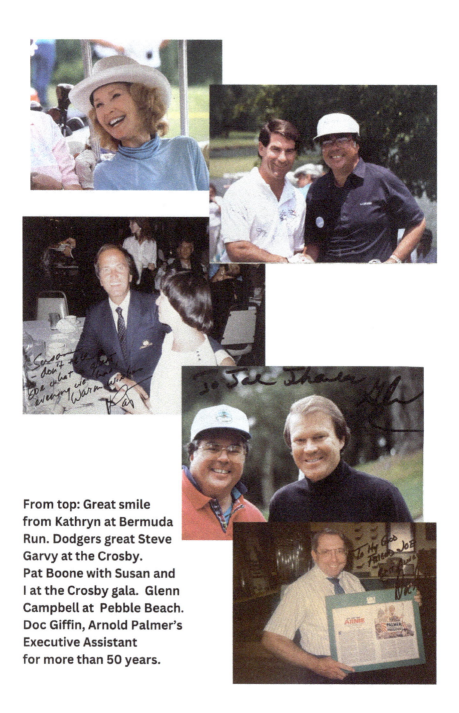

From top: Great smile from Kathryn at Bermuda Run. Dodgers great Steve Garvy at the Crosby. Pat Boone with Susan and I at the Crosby gala. Glenn Campbell at Pebble Beach. Doc Giffin, Arnold Palmer's Executive Assistant for more than 50 years.

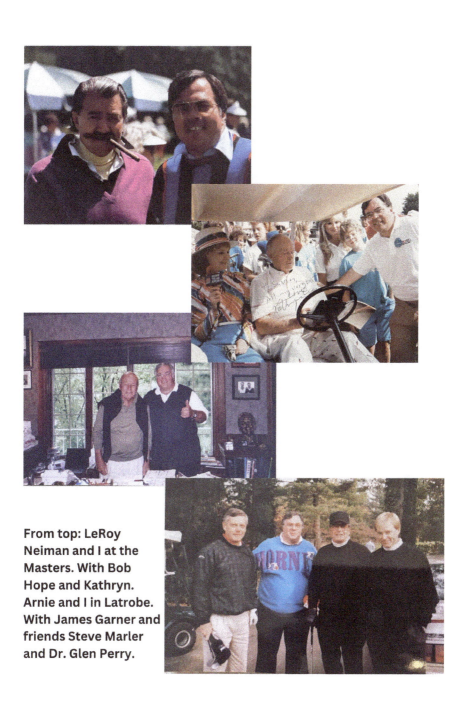

From top: LeRoy Neiman and I at the Masters. With Bob Hope and Kathryn. Arnie and I in Latrobe. With James Garner and friends Steve Marler and Dr. Glen Perry.

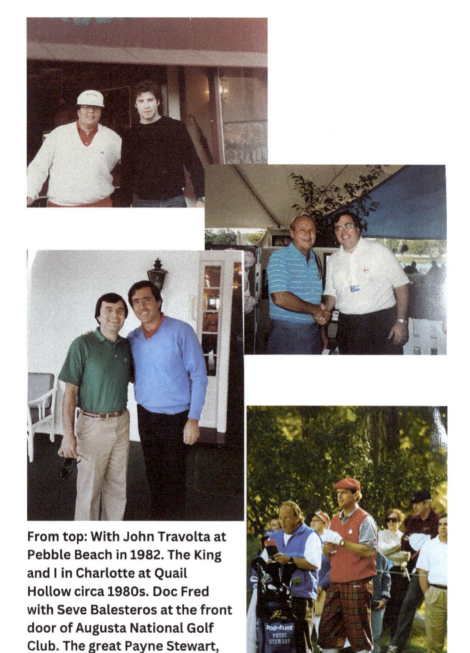

From top: With John Travolta at Pebble Beach in 1982. The King and I in Charlotte at Quail Hollow circa 1980s. Doc Fred with Seve Balesteros at the front door of Augusta National Golf Club. The great Payne Stewart, who perished in a plane crash.

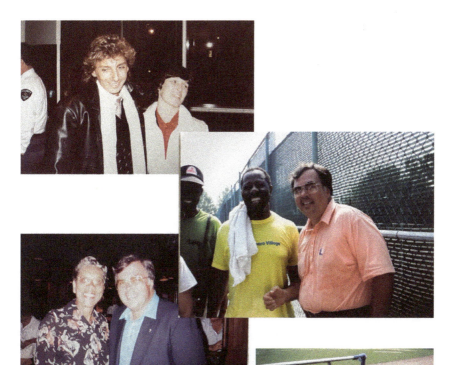

From top: Suzi meets Barry Manilow after a concert in Charlotte. With Hank Aaron at the Lee Elder Golf and Tennis Tournament. A fun evening with Althea Gibson at the same event later that night. Dave Righetti, my former neighbor growing up. A fun day at the Masters with Frank Chirkinan of CBS Sports.

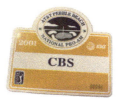

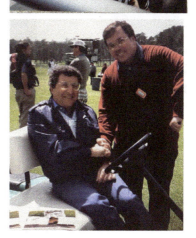

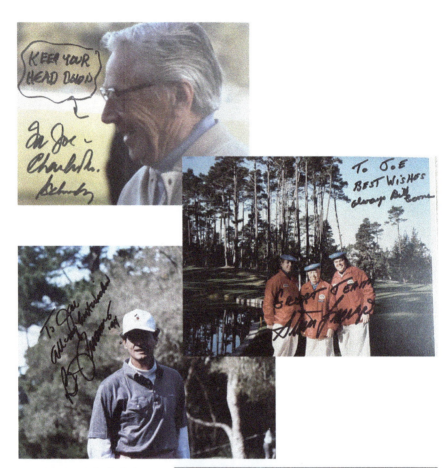

From top: A helpful golf hint from Charles Schultz. Crosby Marshal friends Steve Franza and Bill Coons at Spyglass Hill. BJ Thomas, who was inspired to sing "Raindrops keep falling on my head" by the Crosby weather. With Muhammad Ali at the Ted Williams Museum.

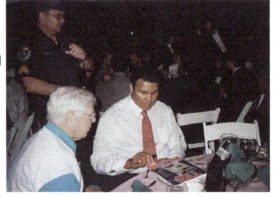

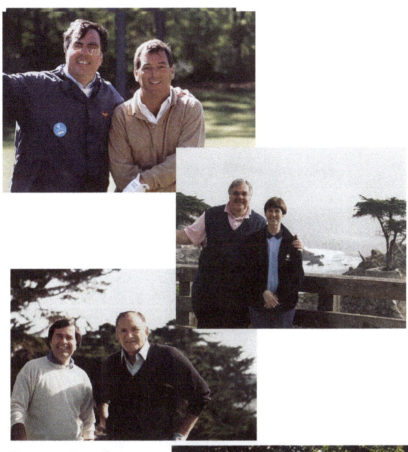

From top: Longtime special friend, the great Fuzzy Zoeller. Susan and I at The Lone Cyrpress Tree on the 17 mile drive. Best friends for life Dr. Fred Martinez and Leo Righetti at Cypress Point Club. With baseball great Roger Clemmons at Winged Foot Golf Club.

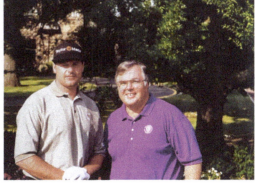

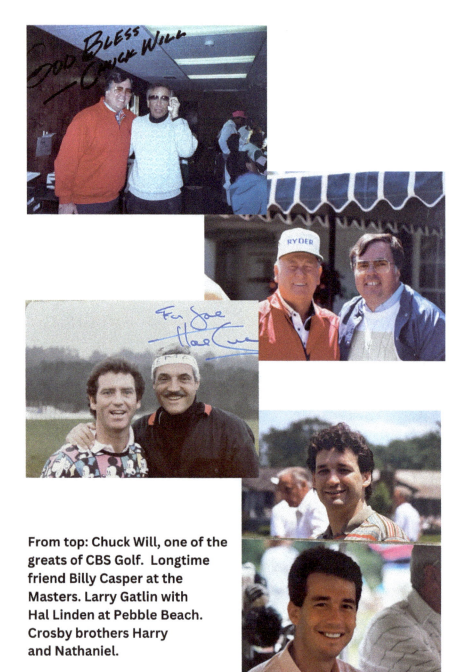

From top: Chuck Will, one of the greats of CBS Golf. Longtime friend Billy Casper at the Masters. Larry Gatlin with Hal Linden at Pebble Beach. Crosby brothers Harry and Nathaniel.

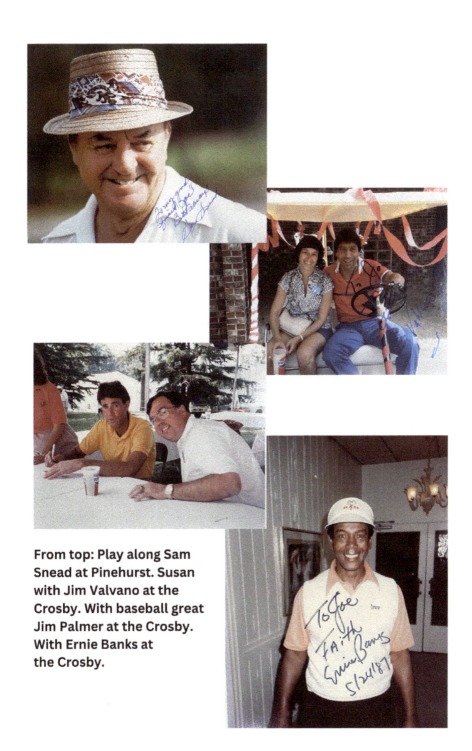

From top: Play along Sam Snead at Pinehurst. Susan with Jim Valvano at the Crosby. With baseball great Jim Palmer at the Crosby. With Ernie Banks at the Crosby.

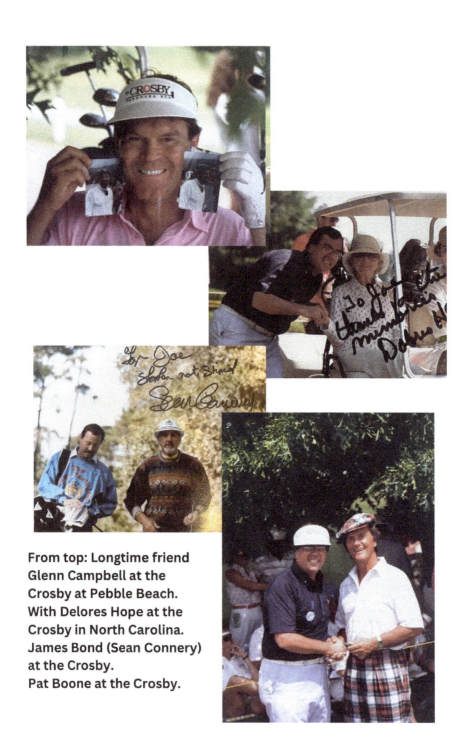

From top: Longtime friend Glenn Campbell at the Crosby at Pebble Beach.
With Delores Hope at the Crosby in North Carolina.
James Bond (Sean Connery) at the Crosby.
Pat Boone at the Crosby.

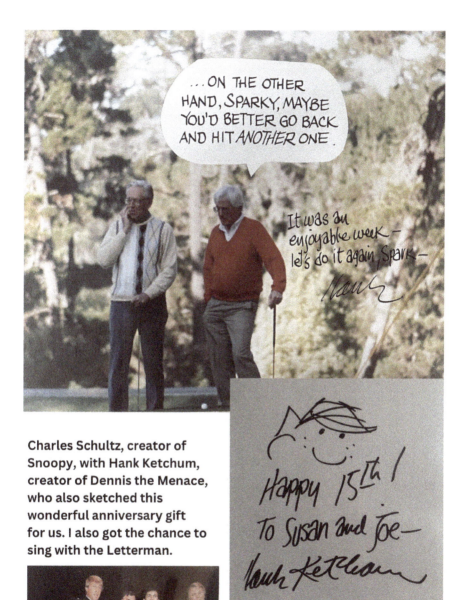

Charles Schultz, creator of Snoopy, with Hank Ketchum, creator of Dennis the Menace, who also sketched this wonderful anniversary gift for us. I also got the chance to sing with the Letterman.

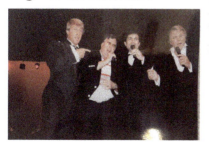

Frank T. Cary
Old Orchard Road, Armonk, New York 10504

March 16, 1979

Dear Mr. Panko,

Congratulations on your promotion to management.

I remember how excited and challenged I was by my first managerial assignment, and I hope you feel the same way. The job of managing has become more demanding over the years, and it has never been more crucial to the success of our company. I am confident that you will carry out your new responsibilities with imagination and good judgment.

You have my best wishes for continued success in the future.

Sincerely,

Frank Cary

Mr. Joseph E. Panko, Jr.
GPD D/872   B/125
IBM Corporation
5600 Cottle Road
San Jose, CA 95193

The Value of Coincidence

Coincidences in life can be a tremendous blessing. There was one that happened early in my career at IBM that ensured that I continued to have a career at that esteemed organization.

One of my roles at IBM was that I was in charge of ordering typewriters for clients if they were placing an order for more than 10 machines. My role was to interface with the IBM manufacturer in Lexington, North Carolina, and order the typewriters as well as all the custom parts they needed. In one particular case, the customer wanted 50 blue typewriters. To this day, I remember writing the color code "56," which in fact was not blue, but actually green. The sales rep from Lexington called and went over the form with me to double-check all the specs, but never mentioned the color. When the 50 green typewriters were delivered to the branch office on Thursday, I was promptly called into my office and yelled at. My supervisors were so livid at my mistake, and the cost and time it would take to replace it, that I genuinely thought I was going to be fired. Instead, we got a call from the client on Monday. He said his wife didn't like the blue paint in the office and she changed the color to green. The customer asked us how long it would take to get his 50 typewriters in green, and we answered that we could install them tomorrow by 8:30 am. Coincidentally, I had picked out what was to become her favorite color.

Coincidences are also how I met many friends and celebrities. The most unbelievable coincidence that's happened as it relates to a baseball person happened some years ago at Turner Field. I took my wife and two friends to an Atlanta Braves game, and we were sitting in the family section, which is where friends and family of the various players for both the home team and the visitors get to sit. They're good seats. They're not real close but they're almost behind home plate. We sat there enjoying the pregame stuff. To the left *of me there were two seats on the aisle. This couple sits down, and they are from Arizona. This is at the time that the Arizona Diamondbacks were announced as a new baseball team, which was going to launch in about a year. To get things rolling they had already named the manager, Buck Showalter. So, we were talking about that. I said, "Buck Showalter seems to be a good guy." They asked, "How do you know that?" I said that I had played golf and had dinner with him and some friends in Pinehurst and had a good time. The guy looks at me and says, "Yeah, and I'm Elvis Presley." And he obviously did not want to talk to me anymore after that.*

By the fourth inning I had to go to the restroom. On the way back, Gene Michaels, who was actually with us at Pinehurst with Buck Showalter that day years ago, walked by me and asked me, "Joe what are you doing here?" We talked and he said, "Buck is here and there's an extra seat, why don't you come down and sit with us?" I went down to about the fourth row behind home plate and chatted with Buck for a couple innings. I told him the situation about this guy sitting next to me and said, "Why don't you give the guy some grief?" So, Buck comes up to see Susan and gives her a hug, meets the other folks with us and shakes their hands and then he goes to the guy next to me said, "Hi. I understand that you're Elvis Presley, I'm Buck Showalter." This guy turned 14 shades of red. He was so embarrassed about giving me a hard time.

One more interesting moment happened when Susan and I were traveling from New Bern, North Carolina, back home and the Crosby Tournament was playing. I told Susan that I had tickets, so we should stop by the Crosby and have lunch and that maybe she'd run into Joe Montana, who was playing on that particular day. So, we went into Bermuda Run golf club, parked the car, walked in the front of the clubhouse to the dining room, and got our beautiful buffet lunch. We walked over to a particular table that had four or five seats left, and I said, "Can we join you?" The man there said

"Sure, absolutely." So, we sat next to, and Suzi had lunch with Joe Montana. She was so excited. As I was getting my salad at the buffet, I noticed a gentleman standing next to me and I asked, "Do you have a seat? We have an extra seat. Sit with us." This gentleman's name was Johnny Unitas. So, Johnny Unitas, Joe Montana, and Susan and I had lunch together.

Taking advantage of life's coincidences will get you far — if you are bold enough to seize them.

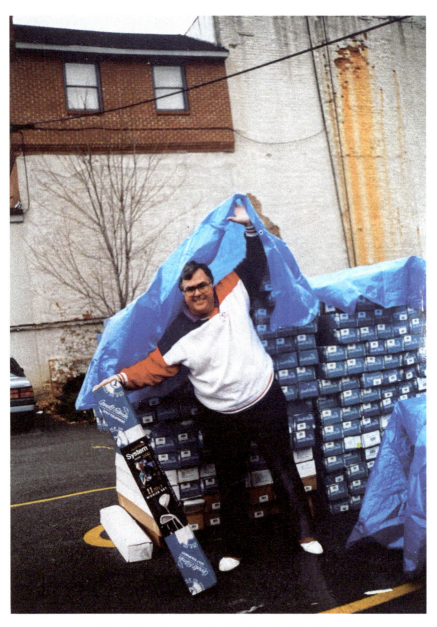

Receiving hundreds of sets of golf clubs from Arnold Palmer for charities.

CHAPTER 5

Lasting Friendships

While golf and my charitable work have given me opportunities to meet many celebrities, there are a few I've developed deep friendships with over the years. Arnold Palmer was one of those treasured people in my life.

One of my all-time idols in sports is Arnold Palmer. I first had the opportunity to meet Arnold at the Westchester golf tournament. I was bowling on the pro bowlers tour during the summer and got tickets from friends of mine at NBC Sports. I had clubhouse passes and I was in the locker room, and I was specifically looking for him. There was an upstairs and downstairs; it was just a huge locker room. I couldn't find him downstairs, so I was walking upstairs looking for him. As I was looking to the left and walking to the right, I turned down a particular aisle of lockers and I walked straight into him. I said, "Oh there you are!" He said, "Who are you looking for?" I said, "I'm looking for you, Mr. Palmer. I just wanted to come by and say Hello. I'm Joe Panko and I've been a big fan of yours for many years." He said, "I think I've met your parents." I replied, "Yes, you have. You've met them several times at the Tournament Champions golf tournament in Las Vegas and they always follow you around. Dad even bets on you and he's done pretty well." So, Arnie says, "Have a seat." So, the next thing I know, I'm sitting on the bench in the locker room at the

Westchester Country Club, one of the finest clubs in the country, and I'm talking to Arnold Palmer. Arnie was working on his clubs. He was taping up his grips and getting ready for the round. I spent about a half an hour with him, and it was certainly a joyous occasion.

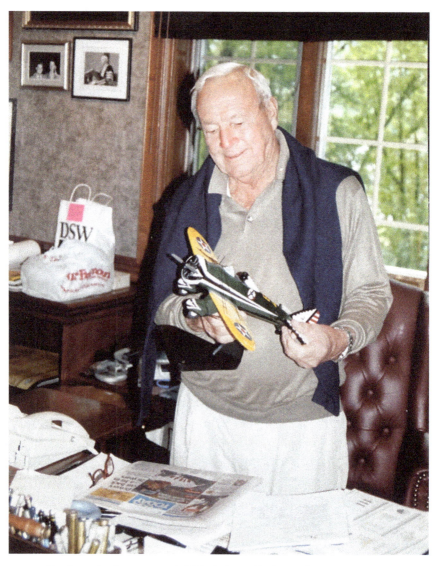

Arnie enjoying a special birthday gift from Susan and me.

The relationship grew over the years, based on my moving to Charlotte and Arnold traveling down to Charlotte with the Arnold Palmer automobile agency, which at that time was a Cadillac dealer. I was looking for a new car because I sold my car when we moved from San Jose to Charlotte. As time went on, I stopped in and bought Susan a car. She was very pleased with Eldorado that we purchased from him, and she enjoyed it for many years. The senior tour came to Quail Hollow Golf Club in Charlotte. With that, I got a chance to go to the senior tournament, watch Arnold play, spend more time with him and develop our friendship. As I collected Arnold Palmer memorabilia, clubs, golf bags and the like, my friend Gene Dikas asked me if I could help decorate their tent. They were having a tribute to Arnold Palmer that year. They wanted to use some of my memorabilia to decorate the tent. They brought a big van from their hotel to my house, and they took golf clubs and golf bags and pictures and various head covers and all the things I had related to Arnie to decorate their tent. Since it was a tribute to him, Arnie came into the tent, and I got to spend a couple hours there with him and his business associates.

Over the years, the relationship that I had with Arnold Palmer grew as I needed things signed for charities. I came to Latrobe in the early 1980s with my friend Dr. Fred Martinez and spent time with Arnie in his office. We got to go play the golf course, which was on a Monday when the golf course was closed, but because of our relationship with Arnie we got to play the course. And lo and behold, he came out to play with us on the last six holes, which was pretty exciting. He rolled up in a golf cart and said, "Can I join you?" I said, "Well, I don't know, sir. The golf course is closed today, and they let us play, but you'll have to ask the owner." (By the way, Mr. Palmer was the owner.) He gave me a smile and a wink and got out of his cart, and we played the last six holes. The first one I was recall was a par four. I hit the ball very long way and I said, "Take that, Arnold Palmer." He teed it up after me, and right out the box blew it about 30 yards past me, so I got my very large slice of humble pie in that particular situation. What would happen two holes later was, I was on the tee, and I really hit it much better than the last time. He looked at me said, "That's going to be tough." He hit it and ended up being two yards short of me. So, I got to out drive Arnold Palmer. A big joke in golf is when you out drive somebody, and you look at them and you smile and say "in the words of Ben Hogan, you are away," which means they have to hit first. I mentioned that and he smiled at me and hit his next shot, 4' from the pin on a Par 4. I had the next shot on the fringe. I ended up making 5 and he ended up making 3. So, he said, "In the words of Arnold Palmer Joe, I won the hole." That was a fun experience.

I spent time with him in Charlotte on an ongoing basis at various golf tournaments. Once, I had the opportunity to work the U.S. Open in New Jersey and on the way home, I stopped by Latrobe. I was there early in the morning, and my van was parked in the driveway of Arnold's house and office. I walked in because the office was always open. Nobody was there yet, so I was just sitting in a chair waiting for somebody to show up. Arnie walked in and said, "Hey Joe, good morning, it's great to see you. Are you moving in or moving out?" Because my van had so many things left over from working the golf tournament.

In recent years I had to deliver some soft drinks that I purchased to commemorate Cal Ripken's streak. I had purchased 100 cases. I sold 40 cases, and I had 60 cases left. I was on my way to Cooperstown to sell the remaining cases to fans of Cal Ripken, who was being inducted into the Baseball Hall of Fame. I was with my friend Hector Valenzuela, and we stopped by Latrobe, and I took him to the office. Hector was so nervous. We took him around and Debbie, Arnold Palmer's assistant said, "Hector why don't you sign the guestbook?" Well, he was so nervous, he could barely sign the guestbook. Arnold was in his office, so Hector came in and got a picture with Arnold and he was just about shivering. He was so excited to do that. That was a pretty special morning. We went to have lunch at the Men's grill, got a table and 10 minutes later, Arnold Palmer showed up with Doc Giffin and a few other folks. They sat next to us, and I started reading the menu, and the menu had a sandwich that was covered in panko breadcrumbs. Panko is a Japanese word for breadcrumbs. This particular sandwich was covered with panko breadcrumbs, so it was in the title of the sandwich. The only problem was the title they put for this particular sandwich was "Jumbo Panko Salmon Sandwich" I looked over at them and said, "You had to put jumbo in there?" Based on my size, they laughed at that. I kept a copy of that menu and Arnold Palmer bought us lunch that day. Last I hear, the Jumbo Panko Salmon Sandwich is still on the menu at Latrobe Country Club. So those were some of the opportunities I got to spend with Arnie over the years. I'd celebrate his birthday and Christmas by sending him gifts. I would always send Christmas gifts to his staff in Orlando and Latrobe. What's interesting about that is I spent an evening with Arnie over the weekend before I went to New York, and he signed a bunch of pictures and a few things for me for charities at his home in Charlotte. I had taken those pictures with me to New York. Unfortunately, on Wednesday night, the plane crashed, and I lost all those pictures in the East River. The warm, friendly relationship with Arnold Palmer was one of my biggest thrills.

The next special player that I befriended by sending him letters and pictures and the like over the years is Jack Nicklaus. I followed Jack at the Crosby at Pebble Beach, and I got an opportunity after being a marshal to follow him one day at Cypress Point. I was done for the day and there weren't many people, because it was late in the afternoon when he played. I actually walked with him and took pictures of him and a business associate. On the fourth hole, he had a good drive and another excellent shot on the green, which is a par five. I said, "You are really pumped now." He said, "No Joe. I'm not pumped, I'm just getting interested." Practice was a routine. He was eating a Snickers bar at the time and there was no place to throw away the Snickers wrapper, so I said I'll take that from you, so I put in my pocket. It now sits in my golf memorabilia collection as Jack Nicklaus' Snickers bar wrapper.

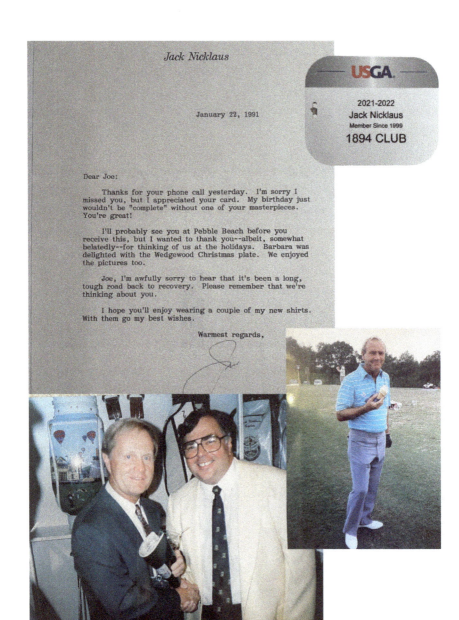

With Jack Nicklaus at USGA Golf House in New Jersey. The King and a cone!

I started sending him birthday cards when he was in his 30s, and when he turned 40, he said, "I don't want any more birthday cards, no more birthdays." I felt kind of embarrassed, but I thought, I'm sending him one anyway for his 40th birthday. I sent it with a poem and the poem read: Violets are Blue. Roses are red. If you stop having birthdays, you're going to be dead. Happy birthday anyway, Joe Panko and Fred Martinez. I got a letter that said you and Fred know how to put things in perspective, keep sending those cards. He's currently 83 years old and he's gotten more than 40 birthday cards from me.

I would follow the family as they played at Pebble Beach and the Crosby in the AT&T Golf Tournament over the years. I got a chance to take a special picture when he played with his boys. Gary Nicklaus was a professional who played with his brother, Jack Jr., and Jack played with his son, Steve. I got a picture that turned out to be extra special, I blew it up to 20" by 30" and I sent one to each of the boys, along with one I got signed for some friends. Years later, I continue to send Jack birthday cards, and he's been a good friend for numerous years.

The other great fun golfer I enjoyed meeting with and spending time with is Fuzzy Zoeller. I always took a liking to him, and got to joke with him from time to time at the Crosby and the AT&T tournaments. He always enjoyed giving me a hard time, too. I recall as a marshal on Sunday at the Crosby years ago on the 14th hole, he had his second shot toward the side of the fairway where fans were. He had hit a shot over this huge sand trap on the 14th hole. I said, "Fuzzy, I'm tired of you hitting the ball in the trap, every year. You hit a 9 iron and it goes into the trap. Hit the 8 iron, and you will go over the trap, you'll have a chance to make birdie." He looks at the golf fans and says, "You know I've been out here for years, and now I've got to put up with this beauty," he says pointing his finger at me. He told his caddy, "Give me the 8 iron." Fuzzy lines it up and spends time looking left and right, making sure he had the wind situation taken care of, and he hits the 8 iron 2' from the pin. Everybody claps. I said, "See, it's an 8 iron, not a 9 iron." With that he ends up making Birdie and making a big difference in his paycheck that week.

Years later, when I moved from San Jose to Charlotte, I got a North Carolina license plate that said, US Open. I drove to the US Open in Pennsylvania, and I got a ticket that was left for me by a friend. One officer helped me get the ticket. I asked where to park. He said follow me, and he takes me to the front driveway of the club. The guards there said he can't come in, but the officer says, "Nope this guy has got US Open plates and there happened to be a parking place right by the front door." So, I parked there. That all led to me sitting on the stone wall as the players came out. I talked to various friends and out comes Fuzzy. He gives me a hard time. And he says come here. I said, "What's up, Fuzz?" He says, "What's up? I had to park in some farm that's two miles away, and your car's parked right at the front door." I said, "See, when you got it, you got it."

In the middle 1980s, there was an exposition in New Orleans that my wife and I went to. On the way we stopped in Birmingham, Alabama, where the PGA was holding its championship at a golf course there. We had eaten at a restaurant that was all golf memorabilia. We really enjoyed our dinners. I was checking out and I was talking to the owner and I said, "Everything was just excellent, but I'm very disappointed." He said, "What are you disappointed in?" I said, "I am disappointed you don't have a picture of me on the wall. He said, "You get a picture, and I'll put it on the wall." I went out to the car and the only picture I had was a picture of myself and Fuzzy together. He asked me to autograph it and he puts it on the wall. I'm in Pebble Beach the following February and Fuzzy stops me. He says, "I go out to dinner in Birmingham, Alabama, with my wife Debbie, and another couple. Before we sat down, we started talking, and my wife noticed this picture on the wall, and it's a picture of you and me. "He took the picture down and autographed it. It was just such an interesting coincidence of him sitting at the same table where my picture of us was on the wall.

Among the other players that I befriended for many years was Peter Jacobsen. Peter was an outstanding player, more of a celebrity in the game of golf, and Peter and I had many fun times together. He played the tournament with the Crosby and the AT&T for so many years with Jack Lemmon, the actor and comedian. Jack and I became good friends, too. Another golfer that I befriended who was extremely successful at the Crosby was Mark O'Meara. He won the Pro-Am part of the tournament with his father one year, which was a pretty special accomplishment. So, Mark and I spent a lot of times chatting together. Mark also is a Masters champion and a good friend.

I've taken so many pictures of these players over the years and I've enjoyed giving them to them. One of those players is Larry Mize. One year I took pictures of Larry and his son at the par three tournament when his son was on the practice green. Larry would put a ball on the green, and his son would go get it and bring it back. His son was maybe three at the time. I took an array of pictures, blew them up to 8" by 10", and sent them to him. Larry has been a good friend for years. He was very instrumental in signing flags and lithographs and pictures for me for charities around the country. And Larry's also a Masters champion.

A major champion and many time champion is a special friend Tom Watson. Tom was born a day before me on September 4, 1949. With that, I've sent him birthday cards over the years. We befriended each other at the Crosby. His caddy Bruce Edwards was an instrumental part of his success. When Tom won the US Open in 1982, at Pebble Beach, Bruce was there. I've got a great autograph of Tom on the cover of *Golf Journal,* which is published by the United States Golf Association. Bruce signed it for me and said, "Joe, we did it at Pebble Beach." It was a great relationship between a player and caddy.

Unfortunately, it was ended by Bruce Edwards' acquiring Lou Gehrig's disease, and unfortunately in time, it took his life. It was a very, very difficult time for Tom Watson. He went on to be a great champion and a big asset to the game of golf. Another man I befriended who helps me with a variety of autographs over the years is Ben Crenshaw. Ben is a Masters champion and also a very big historian of the game. Ben Crenshaw has been another special influence on the charities that I have helped over the years.

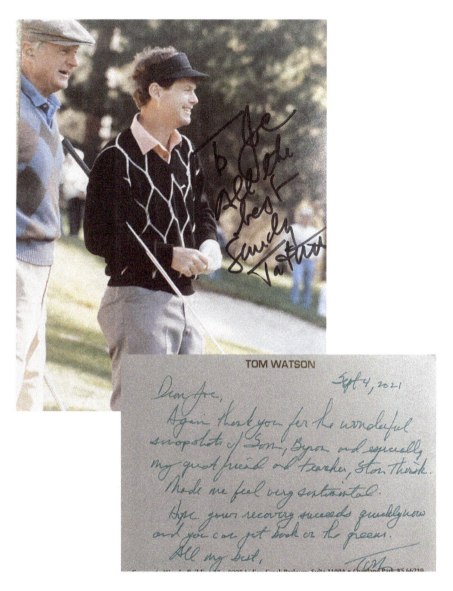

A note from Tom Watson on his bithday in 2021 and a photo of Tom with Sandy Tatum. For the record, they are both older than me.

GEORGE BUSH

December 13, 2000

Dear Joe and Susan,

I am now back in Houston, and I am feeling better and better every day. My new hip seems to be working quite well.

Barbara and I just want to say thanks for the precious Boyd Bears you sent us. How thoughtful of you.

Warm wishes to you and yours for the happiest of holidays.

All the best,

GB

Mr. and Mrs. Joe Panko, Jr.

Byron Nelson

4-14-97

Dear Joe:

Thank you so much for sending all the pictures. Am surely glad to get them. Most kind of you.

Wasn't the Masters exciting as usual. Was surely hoping for Mize.

Regards
Byron

My Wife and the President

Working on the Crosby Golf Tournament and the AT&T Tournament have been an exceptional and fun part of my life. I've had the opportunity to meet many people, take pictures and get autographs of the folks who were playing in those events over the years. Arnold Palmer became a very close friend, thanks to our having met through those tournaments, and he would always give me a hard time about behaving myself, I guess because of my outgoing nature. However, there were definitely times when he was to blame, as happened on one occasion that involved the President of the United States.

One morning, Arnie was playing with President George W. Bush at Spyglass. They started off at 8 a.m. on the 10th hole. I was working the 15th hole as a Marshall, but I didn't start for an hour or so. I decided to walk over to 10th tee and see how Arnie was doing with the President. As a Marshall, I was inside the ropes. Arnie saw me and he gave me a wink. I said "Good morning, Arnie. Good morning Mr. President." They acknowledged me. As Arnie was getting ready to tee off, he was working his grip on his driver, which he often did. He looked over at me and he said "Joe, why don't you tell these people a story?" Bear in mind, there were about 500 to 700 people on the tee waiting for Arnold Palmer and President Bush to play golf, not expecting to hear a story from yours truly.

I said, "Tell them a story? What kind of story?" Arnie says, "I know you've got a story to tell. What about Uncle Harry? Go ahead, Joe. Tell them about Uncle Harry." I played along and said, "Uncle Harry was unbelievable. Arnie, he actually got stuck on a small desert island for six months. One day as he was walking along the beach, a beautiful girl in a wetsuit swam up to him and said, 'My gosh, how long have you been here?' Uncle Harry responded. 'I think I've been here for six months.' She said 'Well, what have you been drinking?' He answered, 'I've been drinking rainwater.'

She asked, 'What would you like to drink?' He responded, 'I'd give anything for a gin and tonic.' This young girl unzips a zipper on her right arm and pulls out a gin and tonic. She then asked, 'What have you been eating?' He said 'I've been eating nothing but nuts and berries. I would give anything for cheese and crackers.' She unzips the zipper on the left arm of her wetsuit and pulls out cheese and crackers. All of sudden, as he's looking at her, she starts unzipping the front of her wetsuit. She asks, 'Would you like to play around?" And he answers in eager anticipation, 'Don't tell me you've got golf clubs in there, too!" Everybody laughed out loud. They clapped and Arnie then hit his shot straight down the middle. So, it was fun to have Arnie ask me to tell people a story. He knew I'd be clean. He knew it would be funny, and I came up with that story on the spot. It was a pretty special moment.

I've also been blessed to share another very special moment with President Bush at Pebble Beach. John McCoy, the President of Bank One in Ohio, was someone I befriended over the years at the tournament. One practice day happened to fall on Suzi and my 40th anniversary, and Suzi was at home. John saw me and said, "I'm going to introduce you to the new chairman of IBM," and we walked to the 17th tee. President Bush was there, and John left me to go talk to the IBM chairman who was on the tee at the time. They were backed up because there were people still on the green ahead of them, so they couldn't play. I said, "Hello Mr. President." To make conversation, I told him that it was my 40th wedding anniversary. He said, "Where's your wife?" I said, "Well, she's in North Carolina while I'm here at the tournament volunteering, but would you like to talk to her?" He said, "Sure, get her on the phone. I'll give her some direction." So, I called and Susan answered, and I said, "Suzi, I'm here at Pebble Beach and President Bush wants to talk to you." She said "Okay." I handed him the phone and just then, John McCoy grabbed me and took me to meet the new IBM chairman.

While that was happening, I overheard Susan talking to the president, and it wasn't a yup, nope kind of conversation. She was asking who he was playing with and how his golf game was. She was asking about Barbara, and I heard him asking about our anniversary. So, they had this terrific, fairly lengthy conversation. My wife was talking to the President of the United States while I was talking to the Chairman of IBM. It was certainly a special opportunity for me to meet the new chairman, particularly since John had told him about the plane crash and the like. When I finished my conversation, President Bush was still talking to Suzi, and they were having a grand time. He handed the phone back to me and I went off from there. Now back at home, Susan had no one to talk to. So, she went and looked for the cat, Ginger, and told Ginger, "I just talked to the President of the United States!" I know Ginger was thrilled upon hearing that. The next day there was a small article in our local newspaper about how President Bush was giving guidance to a local couple on their anniversary. There have been several times like that, that I can now look back on and realize what a wonderful life I've had and what opportunities I've been blessed with.

CHAPTER 6

Family and Friends

That old catchphrase that it takes a village is perhaps just as true when it comes to navigating post-traumatic stress disorder. The love and assistance of family and friends were critical in my recovery, but our loved ones can sometimes play both positive and negative roles in our recoveries, regardless of how well meaning they are.

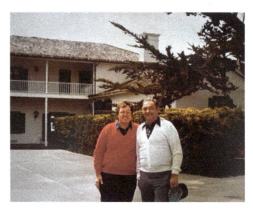

65th birthday celebration with dad at Cypress Point Club.

The strength of my mom and dad and Susan's parents was very important in my recovery. However, since our parents were older and old school, they sometimes had the same attitude of your old grade school coach. Meaning that when you got hurt as a child, that coach would often tell you to just rub some dirt on the wound or to run off the injury. It was difficult for my parents to understand that my brain was broken, and it wasn't possible for me to just shake it off. At the same time, they would work hard in their own way to help me help myself. Suzi's mom and dad did it by keeping me busy with things to do in their home in California and my mom and dad did so by getting together and perhaps playing a round of golf.

Susan would constantly assist me in trying to keep my mind occupied, and she would often give me a list of things to get from the grocery store. Also, if she didn't like something she purchased, I became her professional "take it back person." It didn't matter what it was - whether it was a pair of shoes or even some underwear. I would jokingly express to the ladies at the store counter that the women's underwear that I was returning didn't fit me very well or it wasn't my size bra. Not only did they laugh, but the other customers around them shared in the laughter, which made me feel good.

One of the most wonderful things Susan did was to continue to encourage me to get help from the medical team. When the doctors at Duke said they would take me for some long and indeterminate period of time in the hospital, she was behind me 100% and also would come up and visit from time to time and take me out of the hospital for a day.

I also was blessed to have a lot of good friends and a wide circle of acquaintances who were saddened by the accident. They were always encouraging me to continue on and not to give up. My friends often paid me visits or invited me to their homes for dinner or for an outing to a baseball game. Again, the focus was on keeping my mind off the tragedy and shifting it to the enjoyment of the company of a friend, the enjoyment of the outing, or the enjoyment of the dinner.

While I don't want to dwell on the negative, there were things that people did that they thought would be helpful that were actually detrimental. I mentioned in another chapter that they will give you advise on things that worked for them, or things they heard, or they don't understand that PTSD is not something that you can snap yourself out of. If you try their well-meaning remedies and they don't work for you, it can be detrimental to your peace of mind and overall recovery process.

Finding Good in the Very Bad

It was often heartbreaking to see the condition of the children I brought things to in the hospital. On one occasion, I was helping out in an area in which the children were abused. I checked with the nurses about what type of toys the kids might like. The nurses reported that there was one little boy with two broken legs who loved space. There were two other boys on the wing who liked NASCAR, and they were both really sick with cancer.

I came back a few days later and I had this large towel over my shoulder. The nurses asked why I had that, and I replied that it was for mop up and they would see. The mop up was for my tears, because I would sometimes break down after I had seen a child in a particularly heart-wrenching situation.

I checked in on the little boy who had both legs broken and asked him how he was doing. He replied, "Not good." I asked why and he said, "Can't you see? Both my legs are broken." I replied, "Well, I got you a present that might help." He sullenly replied, "I don't want it." What I had picked out for him was a model spaceship that did everything except literally fly in space. I said, "Okay, I'll find someone else who wants it," pulled it out from behind my back and started walking out the door. Of course, once he saw it, his eyes got huge, and he wanted it. I told him it was indeed his, but only if he worked on getting better. And as I left there, I was crying and using my towel to wipe my tears.

The next room housed the two boys — Billy and Johnny — who were battling cancer. I walked in and handed them each a couple of NASCAR shirts. I gave a Terry Labonte shirt to one and I gave the other a Dale Earnhardt shirt. I told them, "I got these t-shirts for you guys to wear when you get better because I know you both like NASCAR." Billy immediately reacted by saying, "Johnny, you got the

Dale Earnhardt shirt and I'm a big Dale Earnhardt fan. You only got six months to live Johnny. Is it possible that after you pass away, you can tell your mom to give me the shirt? I'll pray for you, and you pray for me and after you go, I'll get the shirt in your memory?" Johnny replied, "I'll do that." By this point, I'm a mess but I can't show it so I say, "It's great that you guys can share like that."

I walked out of the room and used my mop up towel. I often wonder what happened to those two boys and if they made it, but I am so thankful that I was able to give them a momentary respite from their health struggles.

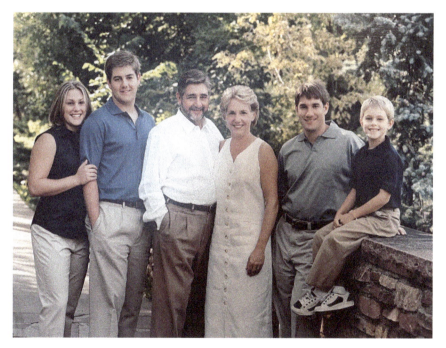

The great family of Doctor W. Edward Craighead, who saved my life.

CHAPTER 7

Techniques for Coping – The Puzzle Principle

After the plane crash, I had many opportunities to meet numerous doctors who addressed not only my physical health, but my psychological health as well. It was frustrating to me as I went through this process and met with, say for example, a doctor who was helping me with my back problem, that I still couldn't get relief. At the same time, I was meeting with psychiatrists and psychologists, and I still wasn't getting relief. Finally, I had the opportunity to go to the Duke Medical Center, where I met a wide variety of doctors, both physical and mental experts, who helped me by teaching me to use several techniques that have saved my life.

One of the most difficult things about post-traumatic stress disorder is that your family and friends have numerous opportunities to give you helpful hints. With only the best of intentions, they say, "You should do this, and you should do that, or you should try this, and you should try that." That's all welcome advice. However, it can become very frustrating if you try those particular techniques and they don't work. The help then becomes a negative. A lot of times, family members would say: Snap out of it. Unfortunately, with post-traumatic stress disorder, you can't just snap out of it or rub dirt on it. You can't really run it out either without getting the proper help.

As I went from local physicians to the experts at the Duke Medical Center, we tried a variety of techniques to manage PTSD. That leads me to the best analogy I've come up with to date of looking at your life after PTSD as the overview of a jigsaw puzzle. The picture of the completed jigsaw puzzle is typically on the cover of the box. The reason you buy the puzzle is that you like the clear image of something beautiful on that cover. It's often an image of something that's meaningful in your life or beautiful to you.

My challenge, and the challenge of many others with Post Traumatic Stress Disorder, is that all these different tools and techniques we tried at first simply didn't work. It's just like putting that puzzle together. You get all the pieces out of a box. You turn them right side up so you can see what they are. Typically, you build the outer edge first, and that comes together pretty quickly because of the flat side along one edge that tells you it's an outside piece. However, in life, rarely is a piece flat-sided, so you don't know where to start matching pieces together to allow the picture to begin to emerge. When combating PTSD, you pick up a piece, meaning that you pick up an idea from a psychologist, or a friend, or a family member, and you put this idea in the place where you think or have been told that it should work. But you often find that it's just not the right touch, it just doesn't fit properly, but you have reason to believe that it fits somewhere. So just as you would with a real puzzle, you go to another piece, and then from there you go to another piece, until you finally find a piece that does connect in that particular place. Throughout the course of my ongoing recovery, there have been different techniques that I've tried. Some of those I tried didn't work, so I moved them around and they still didn't work, and I moved them again and they still didn't work. And then finally I found the right fit and they did work.

As I share these techniques with you, remember the analogy of the puzzle. Just because these pieces fit in my picture doesn't necessarily mean they will fit in yours. However, as you try things over time, and keep trying them in different places and in different ways, you'll discover the pieces that are the right fit for you. So don't give up – and don't get discouraged – you'll find the pieces that work for you.

One piece that was the most successful for me is something that I call the inner/outer mode. It allows me to take my mind out of my body, so to speak, and focus it on a particular item outside of myself. I could be at a baseball game, and I'll be concentrating on what's happening outside - the game overall or on a particular player, thus shutting out the inner focus on my aches and pains in my back and my mental disorder. I am fully concentrating on the baseball game. But it doesn't have to be an activity. As I'm going about my daily routine, I might look at a pretty girl as she walks by, and appreciate what God's given her in her beauty. I might be looking at a flower, or looking at trees, or looking at a particularly well-designed car. Focus on whatever attracts your attention. All of those things get your mind away from your body, and away from your aches and pains in that particular moment. Of all the techniques that I use, the inner/outer mode continues to help me the most.

Another thing that was helpful from a medical standpoint was a variety of medications. Now, I know there's a lot of people who have a negative view about taking pills. The reason that these particular medications were invented was to combat the pain that an individual is going through. Think of aspirin. Whether it's baby aspirin or regular aspirin to help us with blood flow for your heart or Tylenol or ibuprofen to help us with bruises and the like, these medications are all helpful things. Of course, they can be abused, like anything else. But when properly taken, they can be of tremendous assistance. In the medical world of psychological help, there are numerous things that are used to help in PTSD. Unfortunately for myself, I went through many of them.

TECHNIQUES FOR COPING – THE PUZZLE PRINCIPLE

Trying these medications was just like my earlier example of a jigsaw puzzle. You try medication A and then B and then C, and then A and C together and finally C and B together. In the case of my challenges, it took many different trial and error combinations. Fortunately, because I was at Duke, I was able to participate in trials of medications that weren't even on the market yet. And lo and behold, after many false starts, we finally hit the right combination that helped me with my depression and the like.

Nightmares were another tremendous issue for me, as I hear they can be for many people living with PTSD. One technique I used to help me combat my nightmares was to spend a good amount of time thinking about a very successful period of my life as I was drifting off to sleep. In my case, that time may have been junior bowling, or golfing with my father, or a date with my girlfriend who is now my wife. If I managed to get my mind completely absorbed in bowling a 300 game for example, focusing on the 9th frame and then the 10th frame and then the 11th frame and finally the final strike, it would be so engulfed in this particular accomplishment that it would prevent a nightmare. Why it did so, I still don't know. But it worked for me. So that's a technique that an individual can try to relive an extremely positive experience in the hopes of helping to eliminate a nightmare.

The other technique that I used quite often and still use to this day was visiting hospitals and giving gifts to different people or purchasing things that could help other organizations. A unique thing about my background, whether I was selling paper or pencils or yoyo strings, has always been my ability to get good deals at various businesses. After the crash, I often visited a particular Eckerd's drugstore for the medication needed for my illnesses. It was there that I noticed that there was a wide variety of toys for sale that were on sale. As it happened when I came back days or weeks later, the toys were still there. In the process of giving toys to children, I talked with the folks at that Eckerd's drug company locally, to try to buy things on a less than wholesale basis. The store manager cheerfully called it stealing, but for some reason, they put up with me. They had toys there that were originally $20 on sale for $10, and I wanted to buy them for $1. The reason I wanted to buy them for $1 was twofold. First, I wanted to help more kids. Second, I was helping the store get rid of inventory they couldn't move that they could then replace with other items that sold better. After getting this unique arrangement approved by the district managers, I helped these people get rid of their excess inventory by buying these toys at a deep discount and then giving them away to children. That whole process was something that we came up with at Duke in that by providing gifts to people whom I didn't know, it would make them feel wanted, give them joy, and give me a personal feeling of gratitude that I was able to do some good.

What that did for my PTSD is that it got my mind off of being in the water. It got my mind off of looking at the dead ladies. It got my mind off of being on the wing and believing that the plane was going to blow up. It got my mind off of the aches and pains I had from my back injury. It got my mind off of my inability to concentrate because of my head injury.

Giving things to other people was very rewarding. Something I described earlier was visiting children in the hospital, like Mary, whom you met in the introduction to this book. The other was giving back to charitable organizations.

When I went to charity golf tournaments prior to the crash, I would receive what they call a goodie bag - a welcome bag of things that you receive upon check in. Typically, the gifts were very small: a pen from a bank, a calendar, some golf tees, a few golf balls, maybe a few snacks. Nothing exciting. After the crash, one of the things I did to help myself get my mind off things was to purchase items that would improve the goodie bags, such as shirts, golf clubs, and a variety of golf pictures. One prime example is that I was close to Arnold Palmer and dealt with his golf company often. As I did with Eckerd's trying to get low prices on toys, I negotiated with the Arnold Palmer company to get golf clubs. I recall one time I purchased 3000 putters. At that time, the top putters retailed for around $60. They wholesaled for $30, and I bought them for $10.80 each. A charity can afford $10.80 for a welcome gift, and the perception of that gift was that the recipient was receiving a putter worth $60. Of course, every golfer has a putter, but most of the putters that we all have don't work as well as we want, and the latest and greatest putter is always good to have. Since the charity had a better welcome gift, instead of charging $100 as an entry fee, they could charge $125, have the putter paid for, and still make more money.

Better yet, we often had companies sponsor the putters. We'd put their name on a wrap on the putter that said donated by ABC Company, and therefore the putters were paid for, so the charity would make still more money. We did the same with shirts. However, the challenge with shirts is that the charities wanted their names on the shirt. Well, you and I know that if you're going out, you don't really want to wear a shirt with Tom and Jerry's liquor store emblazoned on it. Therefore, I encouraged the charities to not have the shirts embroidered. I would provide say 150 shirts for an event. If they only needed 130, they only had to pay for 130. However, if they embroidered 150, they would have to pay for 150, even if they only used 130. So that was an example of something that I would purchase to help organizations have a better event.

In time, I came to be a tremendous asset in helping these tournaments. Again, another technique for me to stay busy and keep my mind focused on helping the charity do better for themselves, perhaps to charge more money for their event and ultimately to raise more money for the organization's mission.

As I said earlier, the best technique I found to combat depression and flashbacks is the inner/ outer mode of getting my brain out of my body, if you will, and concentrating on a particular television show or a movie or sports event. What's important in that regard is that when you concentrate on a particular movie, you want to make sure it's not a movie that's going to lead you back into your particular accident. I certainly didn't want to watch the movie *Titanic* because of what happens. And I wouldn't want to watch a crime movie with a vivid murder scene because of the people dying in the plane crash that I was in. You have to be careful what particular things you focus on to help yourself.

Taking every opportunity to be with people who care about you also is of the utmost importance. Parents, one's spouse or significant other, old friends, and the like are extremely helpful in that regard. They care about you in their own way. In most cases, that's helpful in combating depression. As I've received help from doctors and friends, as time has gone on, my depression has gotten less and less. Then, if an accident happens, my depression gets worse. Or something happens to me to where I can't physically do what I did before. Now that I've gotten older, there's a lot of things that my body doesn't want to do any longer. When I realize that, my depression is kicked up again. I combat that just as I did before: I take out my old pictures. I look at old letters. I call old friends. I call new friends. I call people who I really like. I call people I don't like. (Kidding on that. I don't call people I don't like.) The fortunate thing is that I've been blessed to like many, many different types of people and enjoy their conversation. The challenge now at age 73 is that all of these people I've known are getting older, and they're passing on themselves. That adds a bit of depression but knowing that it's the natural process of life makes it somewhat easier to understand.

One major challenge with PTSD that most people, including myself, have to deal with is the inability to concentrate on a particular item. I tried to work at IBM for some period of time after the crash, but my inability to concentrate was terrible. It took me 20 minutes to write a three-minute letter. I'd start and I'd stop, and I'd start, and I'd stop again. I couldn't get to the next step. The way I got out of it was when I was speaking to someone, I would concentrate on a particular physical asset of that person - their nose, their eyes, their glasses, their hair. Doing that enabled me to get to the next part of the sentence, it got me to the next thought, etc. It allowed me to look at an old picture and figure out who that other person in the photo was. That particular technique helped me go from being stuck in a discussion, to being able to flow through a discussion and then being able to flow through the content to a particular task at hand.

The inability to concentrate has also affected my memory, both short term and long term. My wife, Susan, who was a very important person who saved my life, tells me I have selective memory. Fortunately for me, I have three psychiatrists who have told Susan that Joe has a huge depression problem, and it causes a challenge in memory. Susan thinks I'm in cahoots with the doctors, but in fact, short term memory challenges are a very big challenge of PTSD. So, the concentration on a particular element, whether it's a person's nose or their eyes, or that picture on the wall, will help you get through the inability to remember and help you focus on what your next thought is.

Getting stuck in my ability to write letters or my inability to remember things was a very, very, depressing aspect of my post-traumatic stress disorder. I recall one time driving home from my office at IBM, toward the end of my career there after the crash, and I got lost. (This was before GPS.) I didn't know where I was, whether I was in Concord or in Charlotte, and I called Susan. Fortunately, I was able to call on a phone in the car and say, "I am lost, I don't know where I am." She said, "Well, just keep driving safely, and maybe you'll find out where you are." Fortunately, it only took me about 20 minutes before I remembered where I was, and I could then drive home.

That particular experience is extremely scary in that the "where am I challenge" as we call it, can alter or set back your progress. After the plane crash, I was in a head-on collision in Concord, and I had the same experience of wondering "where am I?" In this case, someone came across the road in a 35 mile an hour zone and hit me head on. I immediately flashed back to being in the airplane. I thought I was in the water, and I couldn't get out. I thought I was going to drown. Yet physically, I was in an ambulance going to the hospital. The challenge that we have with flashbacks and the "where am I" experiences, might be among what I think are the worst that one can experience in their life.

How you get out of a flashback is a big challenge. It's a situation where you have to get your mind away from where you think you are back to a place you love, which is normally your home or your office. That technique worked for me in several instances. However, when I had various accidents or even after a surgery, I would flashback to being in the East River and/or being in that NY hospital. Those flashbacks were extremely painful, because the intensity of several different flashbacks caused me to think I was in the water, and I was about to drown - even though I was perfectly safe in a recovery room in a hospital. When your life is threatened by drowning, or explosion, or crashing again, there's a very uncomfortable feeling you will have until you wake up from that particular experience. And waking up is defined as falling through and somehow, someway mentally getting back to where you're safe.

Another thing that many people find effective at taking their minds off the trauma is a hobby. Prior to the crash, I was always involved with taking pictures at sporting events, like the Crosby Golf Tournament. If the pictures came out well, I would blow them up to an 8 x 10. I'd take them to the same function the next year and get them autographed by the likes of Robert Wagner, Sean Connery, Clint Eastwood, etc. The fun part about that is that after the crash, it gave me a hobby that turned into an opportunity to meet so many people by giving them pictures of themselves. I have thank you notes from all over country from a wide variety of people, whether it's Fred DeCordova in the television business or Glen Campbell or Arnold Palmer or Jack Nicklaus. The fun of that exercise is keeping my mind off of frustration that the plane crash has given me and gets me into looking at and taking pictures of these folks, and then sending them off for them to enjoy.

The taking of personal pictures has always been very rewarding to me. I'm not a great landscape photographer, but I've been told I am a good people photographer – whether that's taking action shots or photos of people enjoying life. My reward has been a collection of thousands of pictures of athletes and acquaintances, many of whom have become friends. I've gotten to be friends with quite a few folks, certainly Arnold Palmer, Jack Nicklaus, Gary Player and Fuzzy Zoeller, and even a pretty good acquaintance to folks like Clint Eastwood, and Jack Lemmon.

No matter which hobby you select, it can help connect you to others and to the world around you. And next we come to a very important aspect of my recovery, which your journey may or may not share, faith.

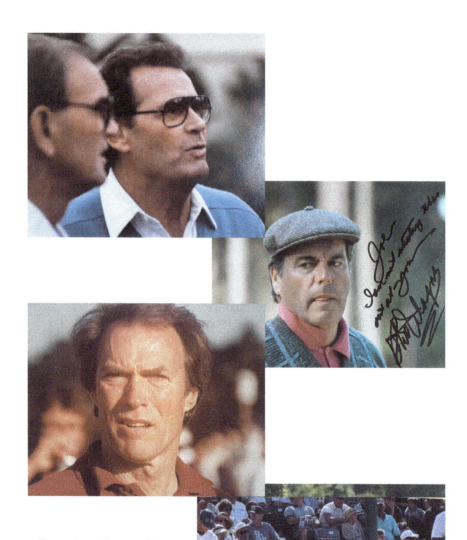

From top: James Garner at the Crosby at Pebble Beach in 1978. Crosby friend Robert Wagner. Clint Eastwood in true *"Make my Day"* form. Tommy Lasorda working hard at spring training in Vero Beach, Florida.

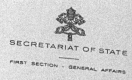

SECRETARIAT OF STATE

FIRST SECTION - GENERAL AFFAIRS

From the Vatican, 10 October 2023

Dear Mr Panko,

His Holiness Pope Francis has received your letter, and he has asked me to reply in his name. He appreciates the devoted sentiments which prompted you to write to him.

His Holiness will remember you, your wife, and Trish Stukbauer in his prayers, and sends his blessing.

Yours sincerely,

Monsignor Roberto Campisi
Assessor

Mr Joseph Panko

Pope Francis responds to the history of the rosary article.

CHAPTER 8

Faith Can Move Mountains

In this book we've talked about a variety of techniques that have helped me cope with Post-Traumatic Stress Disorder. Here is one that might not be the ideal fit for everyone, but it has provided me with an immeasurable amount of comfort over the years, and it may do the same for you. Because of my family background and my religion, I spend a lot of time speaking to the Lord. When you do that, you inevitably find that you become closer to the Lord. In my case. I speak to various saints that are recognized in my religion, and I have been very successful in getting relief from that opportunity to speak to the Lord.

I believe there are three people - three parts if you will, of the Lord and I speak to all of them - God the Father, God the Son, and God the Holy Spirit. Of course, many people speak to Jesus for help. In a comical way, I speak to God the Father because I figured everybody else is speaking to Jesus; He's a busy guy. The father's doing nothing but maybe reading the paper up there. As a result, God the Father and I are very close, and the gift the Holy Spirit has given me is that he has enabled me to continue on with my life.

I have many weaknesses, but I find strength in the Lord. I believe in God, the Father Almighty, and that He is the creator of all of us. I thank the Lord for things on an ongoing basis that most people don't really think about: the ability to walk, the ability to breathe – really every breath I take – my eyesight, all my senses, certainly. In the process of coming back from the plane crash my relationship with the Lord has increased tremendously.

That relationship goes back to my roots. My mother was very strong Catholic, my dad also but my mother was stronger. Even stronger yet was my grandmother. I relate back to how my mother's mother went to church every day and was constantly praying. When I asked my mother to pray for me, she said I do constantly. I remember myself asking, "How can she constantly pray?" As time went on, I listened to that, and I found out. I found myself driving in my car and everything on the radio was terrible. So, I turned the radio off and started speaking to the Lord and asking Him for help for various challenges.

Over the past number of years, I have found myself praying for people other than myself. I don't know if the Lord keeps score or not, but I pray constantly for a young girl who has Sanfilippo syndrome. I constantly pray for friends who have cancer. I constantly pray for people who have had COVID, this particular virus that is going around the world now. I've actually asked the Lord: "I've got people in California, Florida, North Carolina and West Virginia to pray for. People in New York. How do I know that the grace of God is getting to those people?"

"Joe," he says, "It's pretty simple." I ask, "Well, how does that happen?" He says, "Joe because I am God."

When you believe that there is an almighty, anything is possible, and everything is possible. For me, the miracle of life can explain that, because thanks to the miracle of life, we operate with a brain and a heart and all the varied elements that the Lord has given us. Thanking Him for all of those on a daily, ongoing basis has helped me through many, many challenges since the plane crash.

Praying together helps. A friend of mine, Phil Ruth, is a very inspirational fellow. When he knew that things were bad for me, he would actually say, "Let's pray on the phone." And other people would do that as well. Even recently at The Southern Christmas Show, some gentlemen grabbed my hand and said, "Let's pray to ask the Lord for help with my aches and pains." And He always does.

When my shoulder is bad, and my are legs bad, and I can't sleep, etc., I've gone to God the Father many times and asked, "Why is this happening? I am really suffering." And I say this somewhat comically, but what God the Father has told me is, "Joe, my son hung on the cross for three hours. Try that and get back to me." When you put Jesus' suffering for us in perspective, the pain I have from the plane crash in my back or in my head, the pain I have from my operation in my left foot and ankle, the pain I have in my shoulder is nothing compared to hanging on the cross with nails in your hands and in your legs until you perish.

One frustration I have regarding pain is that I'm very frustrated with the pain my wife has in her back. I can't get her to get help from the physicians because she's afraid of the surgery and the like and it's easy to understand. In my case, I had to have surgeries on my back and on my head and on my legs and the like because doing so gave me the ability to continue. So, asking God for help for her and for other folks in my life is definitely a technique that I use and that I believe other people can use to get out of depression mode. Because with the help of the Lord, anything can be accomplished. As Jim Valvano says, "Don't give up; don't ever give up." And one thing that you'll know for sure is that the Lord never gives up on us.

CHAPTER 9

Positive Perseverance

How do you go on? That's a question asked by many people who are dealing with the effects of Post-Traumatic Stress Disorder. For me personally, I've found much benefit in positive reflection. Looking back, it's been more than 30 years since the plane crash, and the opportunities I've had personally and professionally both prior to the accident and after the accident have been extensive. I've found that the most important thing in combating this terrible disease is to focus on the good things in my life, both prior to and after the crash. Certainly, prior to experiencing a trauma, we all have many positive memories with family, friends, in school, that first date, that first autograph, that first hole in one, that first 300 game, that first no hitter, or any of the million other things that people can look back on with a sense of love, accomplishment or pride. Those are things you can rely on as you move forward through the trauma. You can look back at those moments to bring back positive memories of how your life has been progressing until the misfortune of the accident, or losing a loved one, or losing your job, or an automobile accident or in my case, a plane crash.

Elsewhere in this book, I've talked about things that were helpful to me after the crash, but I can't really emphasize enough the importance of mentally getting out of the trauma and getting into the present. Doing so naturally leads us to the good things that are happening in our lives. Even if you lose an arm, or a leg, or certainly a loved one, you must focus on the brightness of each day, whether the sun is included or not included in that brightness. The Lord gives us the opportunity to enjoy another day with our family, our friends, by attending a function, a dinner, an outing, a golf outing, watching a baseball game or a football game. In my area of the country, basketball is exciting for many folks.

I've found over the years that my ability to look forward to a particular outing or some other event has been most helpful in keeping my mind away from the accident. The most important thing overall is to find things that keep your mind away from the tragedy and allow it to instead focus on the good things happening in your life.

However, because of my personal tragedy, I've found that it can sometimes spiral into further sickness or further inabilities that will then bring back more bad memories. So how do you fight that? I find it difficult to fight because ongoing ailments can become a constant reminder of the pain I've received from the plane crash, the pain I've received from the brain damage, the pain I've received from the physical problems. When that hits, I call on the many friends and family members who have helped me through, especially my wife Susan. Susan's always telling me to buck up and work hard on getting better, whatever the problem is, whether it's physical or mental. Her doing so only encourages me to work harder on myself for her benefit, or for the benefit of other charities that I might be helping, or for the benefit of other family and friends I've been able to help.

The most important thing I've discovered is not to give up. What I mean by that is to constantly contact family, friends, and professionals to assist in getting through the everyday doldrums and the challenges of the tragedy. The name Post-Traumatic Stress Disorder says it all in that it's a distress after a tragic accident or the loss of a loved one that we must work hard daily to get through to achieve a more comfortable life - most importantly for yourself and secondly for your family.

APPENDIX

PTSD Resources

There's no one single, all-encompassing answer to the challenge of PTSD that is right for everyone in every situation. I look at living with PTSD as a complex puzzle with many pieces. Just as in solving any other puzzle, the pieces have to be laid out and then put into place in order for there to be a clear solution. In the process of completing your puzzle, you may try to put a piece here and it doesn't fit. And then you may try a piece there and it doesn't fit - because maybe it's from a completely different puzzle that's not yours. But eventually, you try a piece, and it does fit. And then you find where another piece of your puzzle fits in. Then before you know it, you've got the corners done, and then you've got the sky done and maybe next you get two trees done. Then you get the house done. But as you build it, the puzzle isn't clear until all of your pieces are put into place. As you get those individual pieces – which are resources, mindset, coping strategies, and more – in the right spot in your puzzle, you'll become more comfortable with the challenges you endure throughout PTSD. It doesn't all go away, but the overall picture gets clearer.

So don't be discouraged as you go through this process if the initial pieces that you try aren't the right fit for you – keep trying more until you find the ones that are! Here are just a few resources that might get you started.

The National Center for PTSD is a leading research and educational center on PTSD run by the U.S. Department of Veteran's Affairs. Their website features materials on understanding PTSD for those who have it and for those who love them, ways of getting help, information on clinical trials, and much more. Visit https://www.ptsd.va.gov or call 1-800-273-8255.

The National Suicide Prevention Lifeline provides 24/7 crisis support for people in distress or their loved ones. Call or text 988 or visit https://suicidepreventionlifeline.org. En Español: 1-888-628-9454

The Veterans Crisis Line provides similar 24/7 support for veterans and their families and is staffed by folks who have specific expertise in dealing with veterans or who are veterans themselves. Call 1-800-273-8255, press 1, send a text to 838255, or visit https://www.veteranscrisisline.net

The Substance Abuse and Mental Health Services Administration of the U.S. Department of Health and Human Services offers a Behavioral Health Services Locator by location and type of facility (inpatient, outpatient, residential). Call for assistance 24 hours a day 1-800-662-HELP (4357) or visit their website at https://findtreatment.samhsa.gov

The Anxiety and Depression Association of America offers a therapist search by location and mental health disorder. Call (240) 485-1011 or visit https://members.adaa.org/page/FATMain

The National Alliance on Mental Illness HelpLine can be reached Monday through Friday, 10 a.m. – 10 p.m., ET at 1-800-950-NAMI (6264) or email info@nami.org. More information is available on their website at https://www.nami.org/Home.

Military One Source from the U.S. Department of Defense is a 24/7 resource for all types of support – from suicide to peer and relationship support. Visit www.militaryonesource.com or call 1-800-342-9647.

PTSD United has a health and wellness website with articles, reviews and information, statistics and more. Visit www.ptsdunited.org.

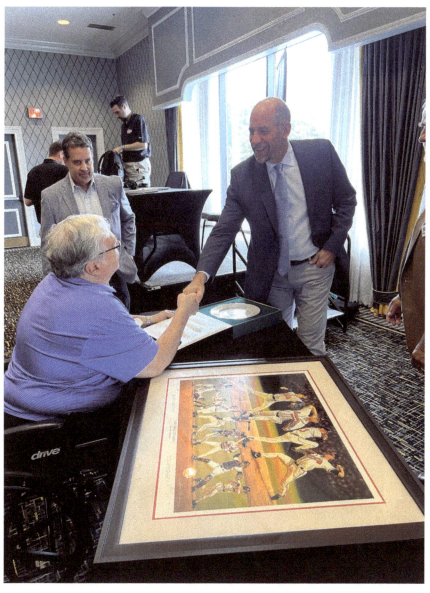

Meeing Atlanta Braves Hall of Famer John Smoltz at the Charlotte Touhdown Club luncheon.

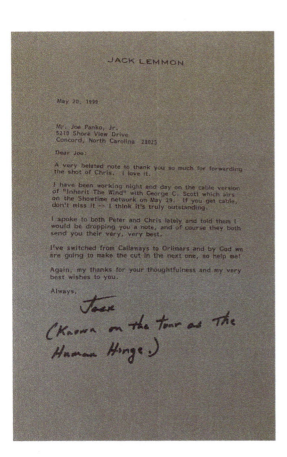

Thank you from Jack Lemmon and a guarantee to make the cut at the AT&T ProAm. Susan with LA Dodger great Wes Parker at the Crosby Gala. One of the annual Christmas cards from Bob & Delores Hope that we received every year.

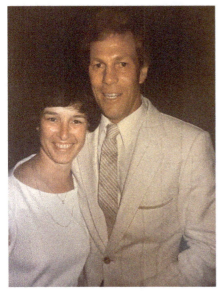

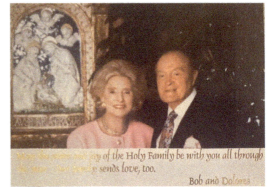

Don't Give Up!

My objective in writing this book was to express gratitude for the opportunities that we've all had as individuals in this great country. Also I wanted to thank all the people who have helped me along the way, whether they are family and friends, a teacher or coach, a mentor for a job, or a team of medical doctors.

Don't get discouraged when something doesn't work. Keep trying other things until you find the combination of physical medications and mental health coping strategies that will work for you. Never be afraid to change those over time as your recovery evolves.

The most critical thing to remember when you are suffering through a tragedy that induces PTSD is simply this: Don't give up. The world is better place with you in it, with you helping your families and friends, and especially with you taking the time to help yourself.

San Francisco 49ers

Edward J. DeBartolo, Jr.
Owner/Chairman of the Board

World Champions
1981, 1984, 1988, 1989
Super Bowls
XVI, XIX, XXIII, XXIV

March 13, 1991

Mr. Joe Panko
Duke University Medical Center
Rm. 3817 - Duke East
Durham, NC 27710

Dear Joe:

Just wanted to take this moment to let you know how sorry I am to hear that you are in the hospital. I hope that you are making progress, and that you will be heading home soon.

Unfortunately, we could not find a cake with a file in it, however, enclosed you will find a few things that I hope will brighten your day. Enjoy!

Please take care, Joe, and let me know how things are going for you.

Best personal regards,

Eddie

EDWARD J. DeBARTOLO, JR.

EJDjr/jj
Enclosures

7620 Market Street, Youngstown
4949 Centennial Boulevard, Santa C

USGA
2021-2022
Gary Player
Member Since 1999
1894 CLUB

CAPE SUN
Strand Street, P.O. Box 4532, Cape Town 8000
Strandstraat, Posbus 4532, Kaapstad 8000

Dear Joe & Susan,

Thanks so much for your recent letter, it was kind of you to write.

I have had a wonderful vacation on our beautiful beaches, and our Ranch.

Have a great 84.

Love,
Gary Player.

Good wishes from Gary Player in 1984 and Edward DeBartolo, Jr. in 1991.

JACK LEMMON

January 8, 1993

Dear Joe,

Just a quickie before I leave town to thank you so much for the photos (they're terrific and Chris and Gina thank you, too) and the original Crosby divot fixer. It's a great memento to have. I had one from years ago but had lost it -- so I truly appreciate your thoughtfulness.

We'll see you on the 15th at Spyglass. And when I'm teeing off, be sure to tend the flag because I'm going to sink that sucker!

Thanks again.

Best always,

Jack

JACK NICKLAUS

June 18, 1984

Dear Joe:

I just wanted to thank you for your "message"...you and Fred certainly say things in a BIG way!

Thanks again for thinking of me.

Best regards,

Mr. Joe Panko, Jr.

2021-2022
Jack Nicklaus
Member Since 1999
1894 CLUB

We donate annually to the PGA in honor of Arnie, Jack, Gary and myself, as evidenced by the tags you'll see throughout these pages.

THE WHITE HOUSE

WASHINGTON

September 7, 1988

Dear Mr. and Mrs. Panko:

Nancy and I indeed appreciated your kind letter and the sports mementos which you brought for us during your visit to Washington. We're delighted to know that you had a rewarding week at golf and that your tour of the White House was most enjoyable. Many thanks for the Arnie Palmer button and the Crosby bag. We'll keep these as tokens of your friendship.

With our deep gratitude for your support and warm sentiments, and with our best wishes for the future,

Sincerely,

Ronald Reagan

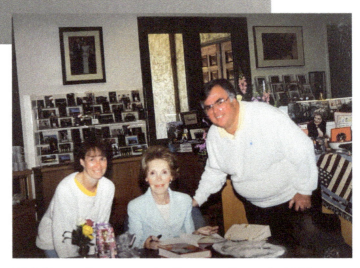

With Nancy Reagan at the Reagan Library in 1999.

Winnie Palmer

May 10, 1998

Dear Sue and Joe,

Thank you very much for the handsome Waterford apple. Did you know I collect apples? They sit on my coffee table and make me feel healthy.

I am sorry not to have been in Charlotte but am so busy getting re-settled in Latrobe for the summer, and needed some down time. Arnie is a hard man to keep up with.

I know he was happy to see you and I thank you for the support you show him, and for all your thoughtful gifts.

Say hello to Concord for me — what a nice town it is. Wish I could talk our Emily into Davidson!

Sincerely, Winnie

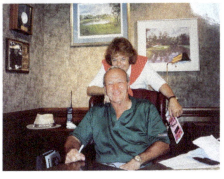

I took this photo, which turned out to be Winnie's favorite picture of she and Arnie in Latrobe.

THE VICE PRESIDENT
WASHINGTON

April 27, 2004

Dear Mr. Panko:

Thank you for giving me the patriotic necktie. much appreciate your thoughtfulness.

Lynne joins me in sending our best wishes to

Sincerely,

Dick Cheney

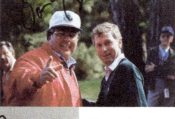

Me and VP
Dan Quayle.

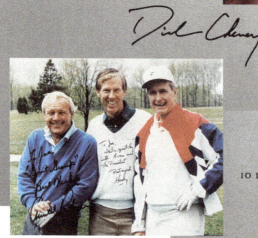

Great friend Howdy Giles with Arnie and President Bush.

10 DOWNING STREET

27 November 1980

Dear Mr Panko

    The Prime Minister has asked me to thank you for your recent letter.

    Mrs Thatcher was very pleased to hear you enjoyed your visit to our country. I have contacted Police Constable David Price who was delighted to receive the photograph you sent and I am sure you will be hearing from him shortly.

    Mrs Thatcher is most grateful for your good wishes.

Yours sincerely

B. M. Cross

Thank you for your kind gesture. I appreciate your good wishes.

George Bush

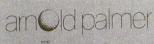

December 22, 1992

Dear Joe:

What can I say? You certainly do know how to do things in a BIG way, and I appreciate your thoughtfulness in surprising me with the poster-sized photos autographed by Fuzzy. Of course, the fun will begin when we start looking for the appropriate place to display them....a new building perhaps. All kidding aside, thank you.

Winnie joins me in sending you and Susan our very best wishes for a Happy Holiday season and a healthy, happy and prosperous New Year.

Sincerely,

Arnold Palmer

AP:qwv

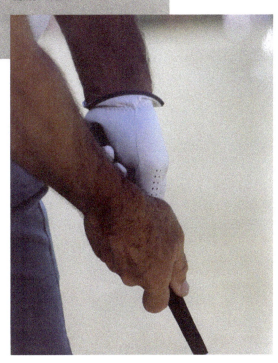

The giant images of Fuzzy Zoeller now hang at the Men's Grill in Latrobe, Pa.

The hands of the master - Arnold Palmer.

ROBERT MONDAVI WINERY — OAKVILLE, CALIFORNIA
Zip Code 94562
P. O. Box 106
Telephone (707) 963-9611

December 4, 1989

Mr. Joe Panko
Panko Enterprises

Dear Joe:

Many thanks for the wonderful pictures you took on your trip. I gave Josie the pictures you had taken, she was thrilled with them.

I certainly can feel for you after your unfortunate airplane accident. Five months ago I replaced both my knees and I will add it was extremely painful for 3 months, but now I am a new man. I feel 20 years younger, have no pain and I say to you that is what can and will take place with you. It takes patience but it is amazing what the body can and will do. One must always have faith in ourselves and in the future.

Our business is going well because we have faith in it and all are totally involved in excelling and wanting it to be a success.

I am sending you a signed bottle of our 1976 Cabernet Sauvignon Reserve. Wishing you the best in years to come.

Sincerely,

Robert Mondavi

Encouragement letter from Robert Mondavi along with an autographed bottle of Cabernet Sauvignon Reserve 1976.

Dear Joe,

I hope you are completely on the mend and are feeling well. I wanted to thank you for sending me the old pictures, especially the ones with Katherine and Bruce Edwards. She and I really enjoyed seeing them.

Best wishes to you.

Sincerely,

Ben Crenshaw

February 27, 1995

Mr. Joe Panko
Classic Art Incorporated

Dear Joe:

Thank you for the lovely gift of the 16th Hole at Cypress Point. I already have it displayed in my home and am thoroughly enjoying it.

Look forward to seeing you at the Masters. Beau sends her best to you. Hello to Susan.

Sincerely,

Ken Venturi

KV/bk

Me at Cypress Point Club back when I played.

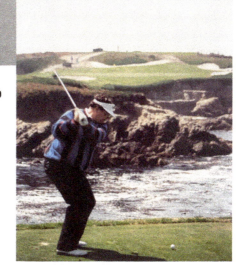

Printed in the USA
CPSIA information can be obtained
at www.ICGtesting.com
JSHW070310190924
69979JS00011B/49